American Diabetes Association

Guide to Insulin
& Type 2 Diabetes

Marie McCarren

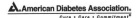

American Diabetes Association.
Cure • Care • Commitment®

Director, Book Publishing, Robert Anthony; *Managing Editor, Book Publishing,* Abe Ogden; *Editor,* Greg Guthrie; *Production Manager,* Melissa Sprott; *Composition,* Circle Graphics; *Cover Design,* VC Graphics; *Printer,* United Graphics Inc.

Printed in the United States of America
1 3 5 7 9 10 8 6 4 2

♾ The paper in this publication meets the requirements of the ANSI Standard Z39.48-1992 (permanence of paper).

ADA titles may be purchased for business or promotional use or for special sales. To purchase more than 50 copies of this book at a discount, or for custom editions of this book with your logo, contact Lee Romano Sequeira, Special Sales & Promotions, at the address below, or at LRomano@diabetes.org or 703-299-2046.

For all other inquiries, please call 1-800-DIABETES.

American Diabetes Association
1701 North Beauregard Street
Alexandria, Virginia 22311

Library of Congress Cataloging-in-Publication Data

McCarren, Marie.
  American Diabetes Association guide to insulin and type 2 diabetes / Marie McCarren.
    p. cm.
  Includes index.
  ISBN 978-1-58040-284-2 (alk. paper)
  1. Non-insulin-dependent diabetes—Popular works. 2. Insulin—Popular works. I. American Diabetes Association. II. Title.

  RC662.18.M365 2007
  616.4'62—dc22
                            2007021814

Contents

Acknowledgments

We are indebted to the members of the American Diabetes Association message boards for their contributions to this book and to the diabetes community at large.

Sincere thanks also to Jack Leahy, MD; Geralyn Spollett, MSN, CDE, ANP; and Russell White, MD, for their insight and guidance and to Jason Iltz, PharmD, CDM; M. Sue Kirkman, MD; and David Schade, MD, for their expert reviews.

Introduction

Should you buy this book? Take this quiz to help you decide:

My doctor told me I need to go on insulin, and I'm freaked out.
　　　□ Yes　　　□ No

My blood sugars are always too high. My doctor just keeps saying, "Eat less. Exercise more. Take your pills. See you in six months." I think we should be trying something else.
　　　□ Yes　　　□ No

I have crummy health insurance. I see a different doctor every time, and the appointments are always rush, rush, rush. They gave me a prescription for insulin, but I don't know what I'm doing, so I haven't had it filled yet.
　　　□ Yes　　　□ No

I'm not the kind of person who just takes the prescription, no questions asked. I want to know: Why do I need insulin? Why am I being prescribed this type of insulin? Would another work better for me?

☐ Yes   ☐ No

My diabetes educator suggested I go to a diabetes support group. It would be nice to hear from people who have done this, but I can't find the time.

☐ Yes   ☐ No

If you see yourself in any of these questions, this book can help you.

You'll learn how to tell if you need insulin. Armed with the American Diabetes Association guidelines, you can approach your doctor about getting on the most effective medication for controlling blood glucose levels: insulin.

Your doctor may recommend an insulin that your health insurance doesn't cover. Some insulin plans are better if you have an unpredictable schedule, but you'll need to take more injections. You'll learn the pros and cons of the different insulins and insulin plans so you can weigh all of the competing factors and find the one that works best for you.

And if you want to hear from people with firsthand experience using insulin, you'll get that, too.

Throughout this book, you'll find excerpts from the American Diabetes Association message boards.

People discuss how scared they were at first . . .

I thought I would never be able to give myself a shot 'cause I was always afraid of needles. Well, two weeks in and I'm a pro.

Was the first shot scary? Yes, it was. But, did I do it? Yes! And did it hurt? No, not even a little!

. . . which insulins worked for them and which didn't . . .

In my opinion, NPH should be outlawed.

. . . and how glad they are that they made the move to insulin.

Every day that I am on insulin, I count my lucky stars.

We want you to become one of the lucky ones: a member of the growing number of people with type 2 diabetes who have reclaimed their health with insulin.

It's Time for Insulin.
And It's Not Your Fault.

You're doing everything the same. Diet: same. Exercise: same. Medications: same. Blood glucose . . . up.

Why? Because type 2 diabetes is a progressive disease. It gets worse with time, and you'll need more medication to reach your blood glucose goals. Let's track this downward trend, starting at a time before you had diabetes, when glucose was not a problem.

GLUCOSE: TWO SOURCES

All the talk about controlling blood glucose might lead you to believe that glucose is bad. It's not. Your muscle and fat cells use glucose for energy.

Glucose can't just float into those cells. It needs the help of insulin. It's often said that insulin is the key that opens the door to a cell, allowing glucose inside. Insulin is produced by special cells in your pancreas called beta cells.

You always need some insulin in your bloodstream because your cells always need at least a little glucose coming in. When you have a lot of glucose in your blood, such as after you eat, you need more insulin to move it into cells.

Before you developed diabetes, your pancreas produced just the right amount of insulin. When you ate, your blood glucose level went up. Your beta cells detected this rise and secreted extra insulin (called a **bolus**) for two to three hours. Your cells responded to the insulin and rapidly took in the glucose from the meal. Your blood glucose levels did not go above 140 mg/dl.

Food is not the only source of glucose in your bloodstream. Your liver stores glucose. If you go without food for a long time, such as when you sleep overnight, your liver releases these emergency stores of glucose. It also does this when your body is under stress, such as when you have an illness or infection.

You don't want your liver to release these glucose stores until you really need it, so insulin signals the liver to hang on to its glucose. Before you developed diabetes, your liver responded well to insulin. Just a little insulin would be enough to remind the liver not to release glucose. Overnight and between meals, your blood glucose levels stayed in the range of 70–110 mg/dl.

IN THE BEGINNING: INSULIN RESISTANCE

At some point in your life, your body became less sensitive to insulin. Your muscle and fat cells now required more insulin to move glucose inside. Your liver needed more insulin to keep it from releasing glucose. You had become **insulin resistant**, or, put another way, you had developed **insulin resistance**.

You may have inherited a tendency toward developing insulin resistance from one or both of your parents. Being overweight and inactive also strongly contributes to developing the condition.

Not everyone who develops insulin resistance goes on to develop diabetes. Some people's bodies are able to produce huge amounts of insulin, enough to overcome their insulin resistance. But you did develop diabetes, because you have another problem: insulin deficiency.

VOICES OF EXPERIENCE

Your health care team may suggest that you visit a diabetes support group. A typical meeting has a guest speaker, one or more diabetes care professionals, plus people with diabetes. You'll find it invaluable to talk to people who can tell you with the voice of experience: "You can do this. I did it, and I feel a lot better."

You can also access a very active support group at any time, day or night. It's the community that posts on the American Diabetes Association message boards. Go to www.diabetes.org, click on "Message Boards," and then on "Adults Type 2." We feel these voices of experience are so valuable that we've included excerpts from the message boards throughout this book. (We've changed the members' screen names.) Here's a sampling:

I don't know where I would find the time to go to a support group meeting. This board is great because I can monitor it between work calls and stuff, and I also like being able to ask my dumb questions in anonymity! The support I have received here has been wonderful!

I live in a fairly rural area and would have to travel at least an hour each way to get to a diabetes support group.

The boards have had a huge impact in how well I manage this disease. The Boomers (of which I am one) are great users of the 'net. It seems to me the "connection" part is the most important for my generation given that most of our families these days are spread all over the place.

Even folks without computers can go to the public library and use the ones there. I've told my doctor about some of the message boards, and he wrote them down to offer to his other patients with diabetes.

I am one of those "old" people (I'm 64) who uses a computer. By the time I had my first appt with my RD, I had found this board and had started reading and learning about diabetes. She knew about the board and was pleased that I was trying to educate myself about it. The people who went through classes with me eagerly listened to things I told them about this board. Having people who have been and still are managing diabetes willing to answer my dumb questions has been a constant source of support.

I've learned more from this site than I have from my endo!

Message Board Terms

You'll see many abbreviations in the message board excepts. The most important is the umbrella caveat YMMV—"your mileage may vary." It means the person is simply stating what has worked for him or her and is not advising you to do the same because you might get very different results. When reading message boards, assume that "YMMV" is present in every post, whether it's actually there or not. Also be aware that people may talk about doing things differently than what the insulin or syringe manufacturers—or their own health care teams—recommend. As always, check with your health care team before changing anything about your diabetes routine.

Here is a short glossary to help you get through those abbreviations and terms you'll find in many message boards, here in the book and out there in the Internet.

> A1C: a blood test that shows average
> blood glucose levels.
> AM: morning
> appt: appointment
> BG or BS: blood glucose, blood sugar
> BTW: by the way

Carb: carbohydrate. One "carb" has about
 15 grams of carbohydrate.
CDE: certified diabetes educator
D2: type 2 diabetes
Dr: doctor
Dx: diagnosis, diagnosed
Endo: endocrinologist
esp: especially
FBG or FBS: fasting blood glucose/sugar
GP: general practitioner
Hypo: hypoglycemia, blood glucose level
 that is too low
I:C: ratio of insulin to carbohydrate
IMHO: in my humble opinion
MDI: multiple daily injections
Meds: medications
OMG: oh my gosh
PM: afternoon, evening
Puffers: people who use inhaled dry
 insulin powder
Pumpers: people who use insulin pumps
RD: registered dietitian
Reg: regular insulin
Rx: prescription
T2: type 2 diabetes; T2s are people with
 type 2 diabetes
U: units. Insulin doses are measured in units
w/: with
YMMV: your mileage may vary

NEXT: INSULIN DEFICIENCY

Years before your diagnosis, you started to lose beta cell function. Your insulin production dropped. When you were eventually diagnosed with type 2 diabetes, your insulin production was probably about half of what it should be.

If you had not been insulin resistant, then that might have been enough. But because you were insulin resistant, you had "relative" insulin deficiency. This means that relative to your needs, the amount of insulin you were producing was not enough. It wasn't enough to keep your liver from releasing excess glucose. It wasn't enough to cover the glucose spikes after meals. Your blood glucose levels were too high all the time.

In contrast, people with type 1 diabetes have absolute insulin deficiency. When they're diagnosed, they've lost about 90% of their beta cell function. Within a year or two of diagnosis, their bodies stop producing any insulin.

MEDICATIONS

You may have been prescribed metformin when you were first diagnosed. This drug keeps the liver from releasing too much glucose. Other diabetes pills make your body more sensitive to insulin. Some diabetes pills stimulate the beta cells to secrete more insulin. These will work for a while. But as you get older, you lose more and more beta cell function. Even with the help of diabetes pills, your body can't produce enough insulin for your needs. *This is not your fault.* It's the nature of type 2 diabetes.

When your body makes too little insulin for your needs, you'll need to supplement it with injected (or inhaled) insulin. As the years go on, you will become more like a person with type 1 diabetes. Your body will be making little to no insulin. You'll no longer be simply supplementing with injected insulin; instead you'll need to supply your body with all of the insulin it needs through injections or inhalation.

SUBJECT: RESISTANCE?

FROM: LK

If most of us are type 2 diabetics with insulin resistance, then why are we injecting more insulin into our bodies? Am I missing something? Why am I pumping more insulin into my body if my body will just reject it?

FROM: LN

When your cells are resistant, it's as if you have added another lock. Your pancreas produces more and more insulin to break through the resistance, resulting in burnout. Now, even though, hopefully, you have reduced the insulin resistance, your pancreas may no longer be able to produce enough insulin to meet even your now normal needs, which is why T2s sometimes need to inject insulin in addition to what the pancreas produces.

FROM: C
Like in a war, the more bullets you shoot at something the better your chance of getting a hit. Your body initially tries to overcome the cell's resistance by producing more insulin. This works for a while until your pancreas wears out. At that point, you have to take injections just to feed your cells and stay alive.

FROM: SR
WONDERFUL QUESTION!!! I recently started insulin. My old doctor brushed off my request for an explanation. I have an appt with a new doctor. You asked what I was wondering and was afraid to ask!

IS IT TIME?

How will you know that your diabetes has progressed and that your current diabetes plan is not enough? Look to your blood glucose levels. Diabetes management revolves around blood glucose levels because study after study has proven that the closer your blood glucose levels are to the normal (nondiabetic) range, the lower your risk of developing diabetes complications such as kidney disease, eye problems, and nerve damage. Getting your blood glucose levels down often improves triglyceride levels, too.

There are two types of tests that will tell you what your blood glucose levels are.

Home Monitoring

You can check your blood glucose levels yourself with your home monitor. The goals for most adults are

---

- Before meals: 90–130 mg/dl
- 1–2 hours after the start of a meal: less than 180 mg/dl

Note: Your doctor might set different goals for you.

A1C: An Average

The second way to keep track of your blood glucose levels is with an A1C test. It shows your average blood glucose level over the previous two to three months. It's like having a hundred glucose checks every day averaged out for you. Here's how it works.

There's always some glucose in your blood. The same is true of people who don't have diabetes. Glucose links up with the hemoglobin in your red blood cells. If you have a lot of glucose in your blood, more of your hemoglobin will have glucose attached to it. Once the glucose is attached, it's there for the lifespan of that red blood cell, which is 120 days at most.

In a person who doesn't have diabetes, about 5% of the hemoglobin is glycated (has glucose attached). In people who have diabetes, that percentage is higher. How much higher depends on the person's average blood glucose levels.

A1C (percent)	Average Glucose Level (mg/dl)
6	135
7	170
8	205
9	240
10	275
11	310
12	345

In general, the goal is to have an A1C less than 7%. Your doctor may set a different goal for you.

- If you're a healthy adult, your goal might be less than 6.5%.
- If you're planning to get pregnant, your goal will be to have an A1C close to 6%.
- If you're an older adult with other health problems, you may be advised to keep your blood glucose levels a little higher.

If you're meeting your blood glucose goals and your control is stable, have an A1C test done every six months. If your treatment plan has changed or you're not meeting your goals, have an A1C test done every three months. Blood draws for A1C tests are done at a lab or in your doctor's office. There are home collection kits, too. (For a list of these and other diabetes care products, see the American Diabetes Association's Resource Guide, published every January in *Diabetes Forecast* and on www.diabetes.org.)

SUBJECT: A1C

FROM: **dd**
You know you're a diabetic when . . . you'd rather be an "under 7" than a "10."

STEP IT UP

When should insulin be added to your diabetes plan? The American Diabetes Association, with the European Association for the Study of Diabetes, offers guidelines based on expert opinion in *Management of Hyperglycemia in Type 2 Diabetes: A Consensus Algorithm for the Initiation and Adjustment of Therapy* (published in 2006). While this is not a list of rules for how doctors "should" treat every person with type 2 diabetes, it is what works for many people. These guidelines are described on p. 18–19.

Step 1: Make Lifestyle Changes and Take Metformin

Lifestyle changes are very important at all stages of the disease. Losing some excess weight (even just 10–20 pounds) and being more active will reduce insulin resistance and lower the risks of heart attack and stroke.

Metformin is a good first medication for most people newly diagnosed with diabetes. Metformin doses should be raised to the maximum effective dose over one to two months.

Step 2: Add Another Medication

If A1C is still not at the goal of less than 7%, another medication is needed. But which one?

When Metformin Is Not Enough

> *Option 1:* Add insulin. This is the most effective option. No matter how high your A1C, you can get it down to your goal if you use enough insulin.
>
> *Option 2:* Add a sulfonylurea. This is the least expensive option but carries the risk of hypoglycemia (low blood glucose level).
>
> *Option 3:* Add a glitazone. The advantage is that there is no risk of hypoglycemia.

Step 3: Start or Intensify an Insulin Plan

If lifestyle changes, metformin, and a second medication do not get you to your blood glucose goals, these experts recommend using insulin. If you're already on insulin, you and your health care team should tweak the plan by raising your doses of insulin, using more injections per day, or trying different insulins.

What about adding a third oral medication before moving to insulin? This is not recommended by these experts. If your A1C is more than 8% when you're on two oral medications, a third oral medication will probably not get you to the goal of less than 7%. If your A1C is less than 8%, a third oral medication may get you to less than 7%, but it will be more expensive than adding insulin.

SUBJECT: WHEN IS IT TIME
FOR INSULIN?

FROM: zs
Just curious for those of you who have diabetes and used pills for a while and then were put on insulin. What caused the dr. to put you on insulin? Did you get to a certain number and the dr. felt it was time for insulin?

FROM: VV
I have been diabetic for 18 years now. Over those years I have had to increase doses, change meds, and add meds in order to keep my numbers under

control. This past summer I had an episode where my numbers were no longer responsive to the oral meds. I was eating around 15–20 carbs per meal just to keep my numbers down to the high 200s and low 300s. We tried all kinds of new medicines, but you would think I was trying to treat my diabetes with Tylenol for all the good they did. That is when the decision was made to put me on insulin.

Honestly, as much as I did not want to give myself injections several times a day, being put on insulin was a relief. I felt so bad walking around all that time with my numbers so high. How good I feel now far outweighs any inconvenience or the occasional discomfort from a needle. Hope this helps answer your question.

FROM: EB

I have been on Lantus insulin since August. It has made all the difference in the world to my diabetes management. I had never been able to get my numbers under 140, no matter how carefully I ate or how much I exercised (not even when I was teaching backpacking to Girl Scouts). This had become so discouraging that I had really quit trying to manage my diabetes. (I have been diabetic for over 20 years.) I had even quit doing any exercise due to arthritis. When I went on the Lantus, I also went back to eating right, and once I felt better I joined the YMCA and began swimming again. Now my numbers hover around 100, and I find I am much more likely to do the things I should.

FROM: jj

I am 49, and have been a type 2 diabetic for over 10 years. I maintained it with diet and exercise and lost over 75 pounds. I had to add oral medications within 5 years. Then last September came along . . .

No matter what I did, my sugar levels did not want to come down in the normal range. Everyone's blood chemistry is different, but eventually your body quits producing insulin to the point of requiring that you add insulin to your regime along with the oral meds. It really has made a huge difference in the way I feel and act. I use an insulin pen with the new micro needles—it is SOOO easy.

FROM: CN

I was diagnosed type 2 about 17 years ago. Started controlling it with diet and exercise, then as time progressed, went to oral medication. About two years ago, my fasting was getting close to 150, and my doctor seemed to think that was OK. I didn't. We had a heart to heart talk and I started Lantus. One year later, I added Humalog before meals. I brought up the subject of an insulin pump with my doctor and September of last year, became a pumper.

"BUT I FEEL FINE!"

Not having enough insulin in your system is like having termites. You don't notice when termites first infest your house. You don't see piles of sawdust. The corner of your house doesn't sag. It's only when they've been there a long time that you see a sign. In a panic, you call a termite inspector. His probe sinks right into a stud. "Too bad you didn't call us 5 or 10 years ago," he says. "We could have treated your house and saved you all this damage."

When you don't have enough insulin, your blood glucose levels are too high. That causes damage that is unseen and goes unnoticed. Over time, you'll begin to notice the damage. Years of high blood glucose can lead to vision loss, kidney problems, and amputation.

Don't go by how you feel. Look to your blood glucose levels.

Blood glucose levels: Normal, nondiabetic (A1C less than 6%).
How you feel: No symptoms.
What's happening in your body: No ill effects.

Blood glucose levels: A bit above normal.
How you feel: No symptoms.
What's happening in your body: Some damage to cells and blood vessels.

Blood glucose levels: Well above normal.
How you feel: Mild symptoms that you might not realize are from high glucose levels. You lack energy. You're irritable. You might think, "It's just age" or "It's stress."

What's happening in your body: More damage.
It takes fewer years to develop the signs of eye,
kidney, and nerve damage.

Blood glucose levels: Very high.

How you feel: More obvious symptoms. You're
getting up at night to urinate. You may be so
tired and moody that your family is thinking,
"Mid-life crisis? Depression?"

What's happening in your body: Laying the
groundwork for major complications and
shorter lifespan.

SUBJECT: INSULIN MAKES ME
FEEL GOOD

FROM: **Hml**

I have been dealing with diabetes for about 20 years
now. After trying and trying to keep control with oral
medications, diet, and exercise, and failing again
and again, I can tell you that insulin therapy (for me,
in conjunction with oral medications), makes me
FEEL GOOD. I can't imagine going back to feeling
like crap again. And without the minor inconvenience of dealing with insulin, I would feel like crap all
the time. Fighting it when the time comes simply
isn't worth it.

I just got my lab results yesterday from my most recent doctor visit. A1C 6.5, FBG 96, cholesterol 96
(yes 96!), and triglycerides 72. Before insulin? A1C

11+, FBG 240+, cholesterol 190, and triglycerides 600.

Insulin is not a bad thing. When you achieve good control, you will feel better than you have in a long time. Give it a chance; you'll see. Good luck.

FROM: TH8
When you said you used to feel like crap, what do you mean?

FROM: Hml
All of those symptoms of high or low BS that really drag you down over time. I would get severe headaches with a BS spike, also tired all of the time. I could hardly get out of bed whether I had 6 or 10 hours of sleep. I had no energy. It goes on and on. Once you get this thing under control, it is amazing how much different you will feel. I know I am not tired anymore. I can wake up in the morning and get right out of bed etc.

INSULIN AT DIAGNOSIS?

Some people have very high blood glucose levels when they are diagnosed. It might seem that their diabetes is very advanced and that they have very few beta cells left. But that's not always the case. High blood glucose has a snowball effect. The beta cells are there, but they're suffocated by the high levels of glucose and stop working. In addition, the high glucose levels make muscle and fat cells become even more insulin resistant. Then blood glucose levels go even higher.

Treatment that brings blood glucose levels back to a healthier level will relieve this glucose toxicity, which will improve insulin sensitivity and allow the beta cells to work again.

In one study, 126 people newly diagnosed with type 2 diabetes were put on insulin pumps for two weeks. Then they controlled their diabetes with diet and exercise only. Half were still able to control their diabetes with diet and exercise after six months, and some were able to for up to two years.

SUBJECT: STARTED WITH INSULIN

FROM: D

My Dr started me on insulin right away. He later mentioned that he might possibly change me to oral meds. I said "NO." While I wasn't crazy about the idea of daily shots (an understatement!) in the beginning, the fact that I had my fasting from 312 down to consistently under 120 within 5 DAYS by using insulin made me like it a lot more. I take one shot of Lantus every morning and keep the NovoLog around for whenever I need it. If I control my carbs, I don't need the extra shot.

FROM: Ll

I actually requested insulin. I had a bad experience with an oral medication when I was first dx, and I was off medication for about a year. Then last winter I got a really bad liver infection that sent my numbers through the roof. I started doing research on all of my options and decided that insulin was the best option. It has a long and proven track record and fewer side effects than most medications.

I had all my facts lined up and started talking with the Dr about why I wanted insulin and she got this big smile on her face and said "I'm so happy you said that because insulin is the best thing for you. Most people freak out when I mention it." I'm still happy with my choice.

FROM: LN

Totally agreed that insulin may be the best choice for many, including newly diagnosed people. Doctors assume that people are scared of injections, and so usually they keep it a later possibility, but insulin has some real advantages over oral meds—it works faster, the dosage can be controlled with greater specificity, unknown side effects don't exist, and depending on the type of insulin it can be a cost-effective solution compared to brand-name meds that can cost $150–250 per month.

FROM: ENO

Using drugs to modify how food is digested, how the liver reacts to hormones, or forcing the beta cells to produce more insulin are a far more radical change than replacing missing insulin or providing enough insulin to overcome resistance. That's just my take on it. Sorta like I'd rather eat the natural carrot actually grown in dirt over the carrot-flavored, vitaminized, mineral-added, nutritional analog. The latter might actually be better for me but I'll take my chances on the dirt version. It's been around a lot longer.

SUBJECT: PILLS VS. INSULIN

FROM: Gm2

I have been doing the T2 diet/exercise/pills and now Byetta routine for over 30 years. And at first it was really easy and now almost easy if I stay on the plan. But I gotta tell you that staying on the plan continuously is almost impossible after the first year or two. So, I've got these "gaps" of bad readings—grandma's lasagna, orchard fresh peach pie, vacations, conference meetings, pizza anytime, fried foods, celebrations—you know the pattern. I've never had a "bad" A1C, always about 6.4, but that may be helped because of the "what goes up big comes down big" syndrome.

My point, after all this rambling, is that I'm not sure why the endos just don't stick us on insulin and teach us to manage that way instead of taking a wild guess about what will happen with the pills, because the pills are not a scientific certainty. In fact, I have always found the pills' predictability to be greatly lacking. Do they just think we're scared of needles and can't count carbs?

Anyway, I'm thinking of voluntarily asking for insulin next month when I see the endo. I think that would actually be easier and more reliable. Just gathering thoughts, opinions, and info before I make a decision. Thanks.

FROM: BA

I asked my CDE today about why insulin is usually a last resort choice for type 2 diabetics. (This was my third visit with this educator who is also an RD and has type 2 herself, and I've been very impressed with her.) I think her response was very interesting.

She attributes the reluctance in the U.S. to use more insulin to two things: 1) patient resistance and 2) physician resistance. Patients aren't keen on dealing with needles, storing insulin, and carrying it around. They know about bad reactions to earlier generations of insulin and don't know about newer developments. They equate going on insulin to failing. We talk about "insulin dependent" diabetics but not "drug dependent" diabetics.

Doctors aren't keen on all the education that has to accompany getting people to use insulin appropriately and all the follow-up visits. Until recently there were no diabetes educators to call on to shoulder some of this burden, and the majority of diabetic patients still have no access to this service. Patients (out of ignorance and/or fear) don't want it and doctors (out of convenience) don't try hard to change their minds. This is all just her opinion, of course, but I thought it was interesting.

She told me about a new patient she saw recently, a woman in her 70s who has had type 2 for 40 years and has had absolutely no complications. She just moved here from Canada and has been on insulin from the beginning. This made the CDE wonder whether U.S. patients really get on insulin soon enough in many cases.

BTW, she doesn't think I should be on insulin, but she thinks I'm an excellent candidate for Byetta. Best wishes to you, whatever plan you decide to follow.

2

"No Way."

FROM: V53

I just received the news yesterday from my drs. and nurse that my blood tests showed I will have to go on insulin!!! I don't know what I feel hearing that. I have been a mess. I cry every time I start to think about it. How am I going to deal with this now? Help. Thank you.

Many people with type 2 diabetes will need insulin at some point. But when their doctors bring it up, many just say no. Why?

Researchers asked 708 people with type 2 diabetes this question: "Are you willing to use insulin if it's prescribed?" More than a quarter said they were not willing to take insulin. Here are the choices people were given, and the percentage of respondents that picked that reason. (They could pick more than one reason, so these options will not add up to 100%.)

> - "Insulin can cause problems, such as blindness." (17%)
> - "Taking insulin means my diabetes will become a more serious disease." (47%)
> - "Insulin therapy would restrict my life; it would be harder to travel, eat out, etc." (56%)
> - "I've done everything I was supposed to; if I had to do insulin therapy, it just wouldn't be fair." (42%)
> - "I couldn't take the needle every day. It would be just too painful." (51%)
> - "Insulin therapy might cause serious problems with low blood sugar." (49%)
> - "I'm not confident I could handle the demands of insulin therapy." (58%)
> - "Insulin therapy would mean I had failed, that I hadn't done a good enough job taking care of my diabetes." (55%)
> - "Once you start insulin, you can never quit." (53%)
> - Here's one statement that we hear often but was not included in the study: "Insulin will make me gain weight."

Those are people's beliefs. What's the real story?

THE TRUTH ABOUT INSULIN

What You Might Be Thinking: "Insulin can cause problems, such as blindness."

Truth: Let's say a person develops pneumonia. He goes into the hospital and is treated with antibiotics. But the disease has progressed, and he dies. Did the antibiotics kill him? No. Antibiotics were just used too late. It's the same with insulin. If you use it early enough, it actually prevents diabetes complications.

What You Might Be Thinking: "Taking insulin means my diabetes will become a more serious disease."

Truth: Diabetes *is* a serious disease, because it can lead to serious health problems. The higher your blood glucose levels, the higher your risk of developing diabetes complications. Don't judge your diabetes by how much medication you are taking. Judge it by your blood glucose levels. Keep them near the normal range and you will be healthier.

SUBJECT: WORRY ABOUT
DIABETES, NOT INSULIN

FROM: **D3**
Folks should not get upset about the type of treatment they need, they should only get upset if their BS goes up and stays up.

What You Might Be Thinking: "Insulin therapy would restrict my life; it would be harder to travel, eat out, etc."

Truth: You might start with just one injection a day, done at home either in the morning or before bed. If you need to take insulin during the day and don't want to fuss with syringes, try an insulin pen (see p. 194). People find them convenient and discreet.

SUBJECT: IS INSULIN OBVIOUS?

FROM: s3w

My wife was diagnosed with Type 2. Today we met the doctor and he prescribed insulin: Short-acting insulin 4 times a day based on the readings and then long-acting insulin twice a day. I am so frightened with this!!! Is there something to be worried that she will be taking insulin at the age of 25? Does this mean we cannot go out, as she cannot take the shots in the open? I am really getting depressed seeing her as she is losing weight and also looks so down. Please advise!

FROM: D3

I just took a vacation. Drove from Texas to NJ and spent two weeks on the Jersey shore. I gave some of my injections in the car. I have injected discreetly in a restaurant. I was a little bit shy too when I started injecting, but now I have the opinion that as long as I am discreet about it I can do my BS readings and inject my insulin. It is no different in my opinion when a mother chooses to breast-feed in public. Some do and some do not. It depends on the mother and what she is comfortable with.

FROM: jj

For dining out, I take my meter with me and test before my meal, in the restroom. Or if no one is around my table, I have tested right at my table! I also make sure I retain the test strip in a little plastic bag in my meter kit and empty it when I return home. You can fit these things into your routine—it just takes time and practice.

What You Might Be Thinking: "I've done everything I was supposed to; if I had to do insulin therapy, it just wouldn't be fair."

Truth: We agree with you on this one, but you still want to do the best you can to take care of your diabetes. Insulin can help you do that.

What You Might Be Thinking: "I couldn't take the needle every day. It would be just too painful."

Truth: You may be thinking of the types of needles used for vaccinations. Those are bigger because they need to reach muscle. Insulin syringes have much shorter and thinner needles because you inject insulin just under the skin. The needles also have a coating to help them slide into the skin. Most people find that insulin injections are nearly painless.

Try This: Ask your health care provider to show you an insulin syringe and give you a trial injection.

SUBJECT: INJECTIONS AND PAIN

FROM: D

It's not as bad as the &@#^ finger pokes. The finger sticks make me wince almost every time, dreading the poke. I don't do that with insulin.

FROM: R2

I was really scared to take insulin. I thought I would never be able to give myself a shot 'cause I was always afraid of needles. Well, two weeks in and I'm a pro. Everything the folks have posted here is true, including that the jab you get when you test hurts more than the shot. I was surprised.

FROM: th63

I went to the endo yesterday. We decided it was time for me to try insulin. Was the first shot scary? Yes, it was. But, did I do it? Yes! And did it hurt? No, not even a little! Now I can eat a little more reasonably, and I am so proud of myself for being able to do this!

What You Might Be Thinking: "Insulin therapy might cause serious problems with low blood sugar."

Truth: You'll be starting on a very low dose of insulin, so the risk of hypoglycemia is very low. In studies, people using long-acting, peakless insulins had fewer lows than people using NPH.

Try This: Ask your diabetes educator to go over the symptoms of hypoglycemia and what to do if it happens. (See p. 141.) Also ask how drinking alcohol raises your risk of hypoglycemia.

SUBJECT: BLOOD SUGAR LOWS

FROM: hb

I was diagnosed in 2003 and since the beginning my doctor put me on insulin shots: Humalog before meals and Humulin NPH before bedtime (four shots a day). I must say that I do have lows sometimes but never of the severe type. I have them mostly around 3:30 to 4:30 in the morning when the NPH is at its peak. I sense it coming and I take 10 grams of glucose and about 10–15 grams of brown bread. My doctor has advised me to go on glargine insulin.

FROM: jl

I, too, take NPH (but no other insulins) and was having nighttime lows. I switched my dosage times and am now taking two shots of NPH instead of one. This has really helped me! I take 6 units in the morning and 3–4 units in the evening, usually around supper.

What You Might Be Thinking: "I'm not confident I could handle the demands of insulin therapy."

Try This: Make an appointment with a diabetes educator (see p. 186). You'll leave feeling much more confident.

(see p. 186)

SUBJECT: LEARNING INSULIN IS EASY

FROM: D3

Yes, you have to learn to give an injection and to deal with the specifics of how the insulin you are given is used. But if you can do your BS readings, an injection is not that hard. Good luck and dry those tears.

FROM: MM4

You will have to learn to count carbs if you don't do this already. If you haven't been to a diabetes education class, now is the time to get signed up. The diabetes educators can teach you all of the things you need to know when you are on insulin. Hang in there. This isn't the end of the world. The damage caused by uncontrolled diabetes is far worse than inconvenience of an injection.

What You Might Be Thinking: "Insulin therapy would mean I had failed, that I hadn't done a good enough job taking care of my diabetes."

Truth: As you get older, your pancreas makes less and less insulin. It's not your fault; it's the natural progression of the disease. You need to use insulin now.

SUBJECT: INSULIN IS NOT A SIGN OF FAILURE

FROM: MM4

OK, are you feeling defeated, that diabetes has won out, that taking insulin is the worst thing that could happen to you? Join the club. Most of us had the same feelings and yet, every day that I am on insulin, I count my lucky stars. And you are probably saying right now, "This person is nuts!"

I felt so defeated when my doctor first suggested insulin. I'd done so well for so long that this just seemed like the end. I tried one more oral med for four months and, with my A1C still going up, made the decision to accept the doctor's recommendation.

FROM: D3

Too often I see patients and Drs staying with oral meds too long because many feel like going to insulin is akin to admitting to failure. It really should not matter how (which treatment option) a person chooses to get and maintain control of their BS, only that control is maintained. But sadly some Dr's use insulin as a threat.

Do not forget this is a progressive disease. Sometimes you can do everything right—eat right, exercise, lose the weight, take your pills—and the pancreas still gets tired, insulin production drops, and no amount of stimulation works. That is when you have to move to insulin.

What You Might Be Thinking: "Once you start insulin, you can never quit."

Truth: This is true for most people. A few people are able to stop using insulin. A person might be very insulin resistant because he or she is very overweight. If he loses a lot of weight, he might not need to use insulin. Some people have very high glucose levels when they are first diagnosed. They may need insulin at first. This will relieve the effects of high blood glucose. Then they may able to control their diabetes without using insulin for a time.

What You Might Be Thinking: "I'll get fat."

Truth: Studies show that when people keep taking metformin when they add insulin, they often don't gain weight. Without metformin, average weight gain is 5–10 pounds. Don't refuse insulin because of possible weight gain. Your high glucose levels are doing more harm than gaining a few pounds will.

SUBJECT: INSULIN DOES NOT
EQUAL FAT

FROM: MM4

You might gain some weight, but it really comes down to what you eat. Generally, if you're on insulin, you feel so much better that eating kind of becomes fun again. It's not automatic that you gain weight on insulin—it's up to you to continue to manage your diabetes with a good diet and continued exercise.

FROM: Hml

Insulin itself doesn't make you gain weight; it just frees you up to eat a little more like you shouldn't. It's still all about spending more calories than you take in.

FROM: VV

I was on a steady losing streak with my weight until I went on insulin (Lantus and Humalog). Since then I have lost only a minimal amount. I feel so much better though and know this is simply because my body is better using the food that I eat. With regular exercise and good eating I do continue to lose weight, although VERY slowly. Probably about three pounds in the last three weeks. It can be frustrating, but I try to concentrate on how much better I feel and how much healthier I am.

FROM: g3

The weight gain is only when you get the dosage incorrect. You will get an urge to eat whenever you get either a low BG or can't tell if you are full because you won't get the BG spike that triggers fullness. If you eat bulky foods such as root vegetables, then you will get another trigger for fullness. Watch your diet and you won't gain weight.

FROM: BK

Regarding the shorter-acting insulins, you do have to be careful not to "cheat" more because you can dial up a higher dose to cover the indiscretion. Having said that, on the few occasions when I did eat a bit more than I should, it's been great to have the insulin to help. Good luck to you!

FROM: BA

Be extremely rigorous in portion control! Many of us have a really hard time estimating portion size by looking at it. Never mind the deck-of-cards and ping-pong ball comparisons. Weigh or measure the food. I was following my RD's plan and not losing weight. She said, "You are eating all the right things—now tighten up portion control." I bought a kitchen scale and began using it. Lo and behold, I also began losing weight. Try it for a few weeks and see if it makes a difference.

FROM: dec

I take 42 units of Lantus at night, with Humalog for sliding scale/carb covering, and 1,000 mg of metformin each night. I have been losing five pounds per month. I started at 20 minutes on the treadmill, and over time increased it quarter mile by quarter mile. Now that I'm steady on 30 minutes, the next thing will be to increase the incline so my body is doing more work.

As far as diet, I count carbs but not calories. I try to balance the carbs (the good ones, you know) with protein and with good fats. Everything in moderation. My approach is one of continual small changes/improvements, so I don't feel deprived.

The exercise is what's tipped the balance for me. I haven't radically changed my eating habits since buying the treadmill, except for switching to 2% milk in my almost-daily Starbucks lattes.

Total weight loss is 65 pounds so far. Type 2 diabetes dx was the "rock bottom" for this little food addict, and I've been climbing back to redemption ever since.

FROM: fha

I've read that diabetics have energy-efficient metabolisms. This means we can survive on fewer calories, which is great in a famine, but not so great in a feast. So it doesn't really matter what meds we're on, an energy-efficient metabolism will cause us to gain weight if we eat more than we burn, and we burn slower than most. It helps me to think of it that way.

3

Insulins

Before you developed diabetes, your body produced a low level of insulin all day and all night.
This is called **basal** or background insulin. When
you ate, your body produced extra insulin, or a
bolus. The pattern of the bolus depended on how
big your meal was and what types of food you ate.

Your Insulin Levels Before You Developed Diabetes

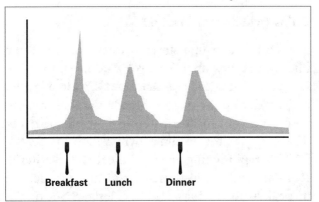

Breakfast   Lunch   Dinner

If your blood glucose levels are too high, your pancreas is not producing enough basal insulin, or it's not producing enough insulin after meals, or both. You can make up for these shortages by supplementing with injected (or inhaled) insulin.

TYPES OF INSULINS

Basal Insulin

A good basal insulin provides a low, steady amount of insulin activity. It also has a long **duration**. It lasts at least half a day to as long as 24 hours, so you'll need to take it only once or twice a day.

Two insulins meet these criteria: glargine and detemir. Another insulin used for basal coverage is NPH. NPH does have a peak, but it's very broad. We discuss the pros and cons of these three insulins on p. 67–70.

Bolus (Mealtime) Insulin

A good bolus insulin starts to work soon after you inject it (a quick **onset**), so you can take it right before you eat. It also has a sharp **peak**: a lot of insulin activity during the two to three hours that the glucose from your meal is entering your bloodstream. Then, ideally, the insulin activity will drop off.

The rapid-acting insulins meet these criteria. Regular insulin is also used for meal coverage, but its peak is not as sharp and lasts longer. See p. 87.

Action Profiles of Insulins

	Onset	Peak	Duration
Mealtime (Bolus) Insulins			
Rapid-acting, injected (aspart, lispro, and glulisine)	less than 15 minutes	1–2 hours	3–4 hours
Rapid-acting, inhaled (inhaled dry, powdered insulin)	less than 15 minutes	30–90 minutes	6 hours
Regular	30 minutes to 1 hour	2–3 hours	3–6 hours
Basal Insulins			
NPH		4–10 hours	10–16 hours
Detemir		fairly flat	12 hours with low doses, over 20 hours with high doses
Glargine		fairly flat	20–24 hours

Action Curves of Insulins

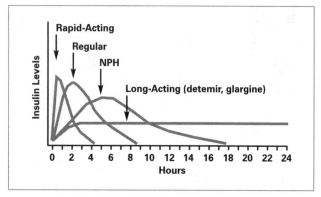

Insulin: Onset, Peak, and Duration

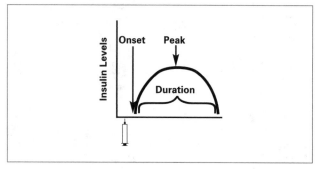

Onset: How soon after injection the insulin begins lowering blood glucose. Also known as lag time.

Peak: When the insulin is lowering your blood glucose levels the most. It's important to know the onset and peak for your mealtime insulin so you know when to take it.

Duration: The total time the insulin lowers your blood glucose.

MANUFACTURED INSULINS

Years ago, people used animal insulins. Today, we use "human" insulin and the insulin analogs.

Human insulin is made in labs. The genetic code for human insulin is inserted into bacteria or yeast so they produce human insulin. Different additives in human insulin produce different action profiles.

The insulin analogs—aspart, lispro, glulisine, glargine, and detemir—are the newer insulins. They're like human insulin but with small changes in the chemical structure. These changes produce insulins with different action profiles. Insulin analogs are also made in labs. They require a prescription. Some insurance plans cover the older insulins but not the insulin analogs, which are more expensive.

Insulins Available in the U.S.

Type	Generic Name	Brand Name	Made by	Website
Used for				
Rapid-Acting	aspart	NovoLog	Novo Nordisk	www.novolog.com
Meals	glulisine	Apidra	Sanofi-Aventis	www.apidra.com
(bolus)	lispro	Humalog	Lilly	www.humalog.com
	regular inhaled	Exubera	Pfizer	www.exubera.com
Regular	regular	Humulin R	Lilly	
Meals	regular	Novolin R	Novo Nordisk	
(bolus)				
NPH	NPH	Humulin N	Lilly	
basal only	NPH	Novolin N	Novo Nordisk	
or basal				
+ meal				
(bolus)				

Long-Acting *Basal*	glargine detemir	Lantus Levemir	Sanofi-Aventis Novo Nordisk	www.lantus.com www.levemir-us.com
Premixed *meal (bolus) + basal*	75% delayed lispro 25% lispro	Humalog Mix 75/25	Lilly	www.humalog.com
	50% delayed lispro 50% lispro	Humalog Mix 50/50	Lilly	www.humalog.com
	70% NPH 30% regular	Humulin 70/30	Lilly	
	50% NPH 50% regular	Humulin 50/50	Lilly	
	70% delayed aspart 30% aspart	NovoLog Mix 70/30*	Novo Nordisk	www.novologmix70-30.com
	70% NPH 30% regular	Novolin 70/30*	Novo Nordisk	

*Note the difference between Novolin 70/30 (30% regular) versus NovoLog 70/30 (30% rapid-acting aspart).

Premixed Insulin

Although people talk about premixes as though they contain two insulins, it's really just one insulin. A binding agent is added to rapid-acting or regular insulin. This makes some of the insulin (75%, 70%, or 50%) intermediate acting. People often refer to this part as "NPH." You inject a premix before a meal. You get a peak from the rapid-acting or regular portion and then a long trailing off that gives basal coverage.

Cloudy Insulins: Rock 'n' Roll

NPH and the premixed insulins are normally cloudy. These insulins settle when they sit around, like orange juice that sits in your refrigerator. You have to gently remix any cloudy insulin every time before you use it. If you don't, the doses you draw will be different from each other and will give unpredictable results.

- Gently roll the bottle or insulin pen between your hands 10 times and turn it upside down 10 times.
- Don't shake it! Shaking makes bubbles, and then your dose won't be right.

TIMING OF REGULAR INSULIN

It normally takes only about 10 minutes for food that you eat to start to be digested, to be absorbed, and to turn up as glucose in your blood. But it takes about 30 minutes after injection for regular insulin to start to lower blood glucose. If you inject regular insulin right before you eat, your blood glucose level will go too high, until the insulin catches up.

The general rule is to inject regular insulin (or a premix that contains regular) 30 minutes before you start to eat. This is often inconvenient, so most doctors and patients favor rapid-acting insulins. Typically, you take rapid-acting insulin right before you eat. This is more convenient, and it becomes even more important when you can't predict or control when your food will come, such as at a restaurant.

If you do use regular insulin or a premix that contains regular, you may want to try the timing chart on p. 54, which has been used for many years by people with type 1 diabetes.

Check Your Blood Glucose Level 45 Minutes Before Meal. If It Is:	Right Away:	Inject Regular Insulin (or a Mix that Contains Regular):
below 50 mg/dl	eat or drink something with sugar	when finishing the meal
50–70 mg/dl	eat or drink something with sugar	at mealtime
70–120 mg/dl		15 minutes before the meal
120–180 mg/dl		30 minutes before the meal
over 180 mg/dl		45 minutes before the meal

WHEN TO TAKE REGULAR INSULIN

FROM: wt

I've been on metformin and glyburide. Now, I've had some high blood sugar levels . . . one was 334 and another was 287. I took some regular insulin and one time it brought me down to 47. I took the insulin about 3 hours after I had eaten. Is this the wrong time to take insulin? If so, when is the right time?

FROM: tm

Wow! I'm upset that a doctor would prescribe insulin to you and not tell you when and how much to take! You need to call that doctor back and get directions from him or her. Regular insulin needs to be taken about a half hour BEFORE eating.

Slow Stomach

Some people with diabetes develop a condition called gastroparesis. Food moves from the stomach to the intestines more slowly than normal and at unpredictable times. This can lead to unpredictable highs and lows in blood glucose levels. People with severe gastroparesis have symptoms such as bloating, nausea, or vomiting. Those with mild gastroparesis may not have these symptoms, but their blood glucose levels may still be affected.

- Regular insulin, with its broader peak, may work better than the sharper spike of rapid-acting insulin if you have gastroparesis.
- Some people with gastroparesis find rapid-acting works better for them. They don't take the insulin before the meal. They check their blood glucose levels after they eat and inject rapid-acting insulin when their blood glucose starts to rise.

INHALED INSULIN

Exubera is the first inhaled insulin to reach the market. It's regular insulin, but it acts like a rapid-acting insulin. It covers meals. It doesn't cover your basal insulin needs.

You shouldn't use Exubera if you smoke or have smoked in the last 6 months or have lung problems (for example, asthma, chronic obstructive pulmonary disease, or emphysema).

Using Exubera

Your lung function should be tested before you start Exubera. This is done with spirometry. You take a deep breath and blow into a tube as hard as you can. This test should be done again 6 and 12 months after you start using Exubera.

Exubera comes in blister packs with either 1-mg or 3-mg doses. A 1-mg blister is equal to about 3 units of injected regular insulin. A 3-mg blister is equal to about 8 units. Combine blister sizes to use the fewest blisters possible. For example, if you need 4 mg of inhaled insulin, use a 3-mg and a 1-mg blister rather than four 1-mg blisters.

You take Exubera 10 minutes before you eat. When you're new to Exubera, you might cough within seconds or minutes after using it. This usually happens less as you keep using it. If you develop a longer-lasting cough or wheezing or if you find yourself often short of breath, your lung function should be tested more often. You can expect to lose a little bit of lung function, but you shouldn't notice this in your everyday life. If you lose anything more than that, then you'll need to stop using Exubera.

SUBJECT: AM I THE ONLY ONE ON EXUBERA?

FROM: **Rk**

Still feeling like the only person in the world on Exubera, but I still love it. Tomorrow will be the end of the first week. Inhaled insulin is SOOOOO cool! I just wish I could find ANYONE in the world out there also on it. I have been to a hundred different websites looking, but so far no luck finding someone else. Had a funny thing happen today: I was at work, and they referred to my inhaler as my "insulin bong."

Actually I was scared at how big I THOUGHT it would be. It is not that large. It collapses for storage. I keep mine in my purse, inside a quart-size plastic bag, and when collapsed, it fits in that perfectly. Well, point anyone my way if you find anyone asking about this. I read the board everyday in hopes that one day I will find an Exubera buddy.

FROM: Psp
Does it leave any taste in your mouth? Sore throat? Any type of after effect?

FROM: Rk
Actually, no there is no taste during or afterwards. Only thing I have noticed is that if I inhale too quickly or forcefully the powder hits the back of my throat and tickles, so I end up coughing, but it is my error. I am supposed to inhale it by breathing normally. No sore throat or really any negative side effects. It is amazing just how fast it works, too. Been testing my little fingers to death! I feel really fortunate to be on this now. It is such a big leap forward in the treatment of diabetes, especially for those with needle phobia.

FROM: hg
I saw my endo today and am starting Exubera after a pulmonary function test next week.

FROM: Rk
Good luck with the test. It's easy, just breathe into a tube and keep pushing that breath out as long as you honestly can . . . then push just a little more!

DO YOU NEED CONCENTRATED INSULIN?

If you're using more than 200 units of insulin a day
and are still not reaching your blood glucose goals,
your body is very resistant to insulin. Such extreme
insulin resistance is seen in people with certain rare
forms of diabetes, in some people with type 2 diabetes who are obese, and temporarily in some
people during pregnancy, infection, or steroid use.
You might want to ask your doctor about switching
to concentrated insulin.

The concentration of every insulin listed on p.
50–51 is U-100. They have 100 units of insulin per
milliliter of liquid. There is only one concentrated
insulin sold in the U.S.: U-500 Humulin R. It has
500 units of insulin per milliliter of liquid. Although
U-500 is regular insulin, its action profile (peak
and duration) is more like that of NPH than of
U-100 regular insulin.

U-500 comes in 20-ml vials. These cost more than twice as much as a 10-ml vial of U-100, but when you figure out the cost per unit of insulin, it's less expensive.

Few doctors are familiar with U-500. Researchers at the National Institute of Diabetes and Digestive and Kidney Diseases have developed guidelines for making the switch from U-100 to U-500. They are as follows:

Add up all the doses of insulin you take in a day. If your daily insulin dose is:

200–300 units
- Switch to U-500 twice a day: before breakfast and before dinner.
- This will be your only insulin.

300–750 units
- Switch to U-500 three times a day: before breakfast, lunch, and dinner.

750–2,000 units
- Switch to U-500 four times a day: before breakfast, lunch, dinner, and bedtime.
- The bedtime dose is slightly smaller.

More than 2,000 units
- U-500 four times a day, as above.
- Inject no more than 500 units at any one site. For example, if you take 700 units for

---

one dose, inject 350 units in one area and 350 units in a different spot at least one inch away.

Check your blood glucose levels before breakfast and before dinner. Your goal in the morning is 70–120 mg/dl. Look for patterns: highs or lows at the same time of day for several days.

- If your morning glucose levels are less than 70 mg/dl, reduce your last insulin dose of the day (either the dinner or bedtime dose).
- If your morning glucose levels are above your goal, raise all your doses of U-500.

U-500 is available by prescription only. Your pharmacy will have to special order it, and it may take a day or two. Ask your doctor to write the prescription in units and in volume and to tell you what that looks like on your U-100 syringe. Review the instructions with your pharmacist when you pick up the prescription. For example, if you need 150 units three times a day, the prescription might be written as: "Regular Insulin U-500, 150 units, inject 0.3 ml subcutaneously (under the skin) three times daily before meals." On your U-100 syringe, you will need to draw up what looks like 30 units, but it will really be 150 units because U-500 is five times as strong as U-100.

4

Starting Insulin
What's the Best Way?

If you go to a meeting for diabetes specialists, there will likely be a talk on starting insulin therapy in people with type 2 diabetes.

The first speaker will argue eloquently in favor of one plan. She'll display the results of study after study that show that this insulin plan works well. She'll say how well she has seen this work in her own patients.

The second speaker will get up and argue just as persuasively that a different plan is the one to use. Again, study results and case studies.

But the debate is friendly because, in the end, both speakers agree on these points:

- Too many people with type 2 diabetes delay going on insulin for far too long.
- The important thing is to get on any reasonable insulin plan as soon as you need it.

- Whichever plan you start with, don't pull your punches. Keep raising the doses until your blood glucose levels are to your goal.

"WHAT ABOUT MY DIABETES PILLS?"

If you stopped taking your other diabetes medications and used only insulin, you'd need high doses of insulin (80–100 units a day) to control your blood glucose levels and you'd probably gain weight. So your doctor will probably have you keep taking one or two of your other diabetes medications and add insulin. You'll use less insulin, have better blood glucose control, and see less weight gain.

The table on p. 65 describes many of the classes of diabetes pills and possible results that arise when they are combined with insulin.

Class of Diabetes Pill *Examples*	Main Action	Advantages When Used with Insulin vs. Using Insulin Alone	Possible Problems When Used with Insulin
Biguanide *metformin*	Keeps liver from releasing glucose	• Better A1C with lower doses of insulin. • Often no weight gain.	
Sulfonylureas *glipizide, glyburide, glimepiride*	Spur pancreas to produce insulin	• Your own pancreas, helped by the sulfonylurea, may be able to cover meals.	
Glitazones (thiazolidinediones) *Actos, Avandia*	Make muscle cells more sensitive to insulin	• Less available data than other oral medications. • Can allow much lower doses of insulin. • May need to lower the dose of the glitazone.	Fluid retention, increasing risk of congestive heart failure, weight gain
Meglitinides *Starlix, Prandin*	Spur pancreas to produce insulin	Too little data available	Too little data available

ONE INSULIN OR TWO?

If you're starting insulin when you first need it, you probably need only basal insulin. But if you and your doctor have waited until your diabetes is further along, you will need both basal and mealtime insulins.

If your A1C is less than 8.5%, there's a good chance you need only basal insulin at this time.

BUT

If your A1C is over 8.5%, you may need basal and mealtime insulin.

- Your doctor may start you on basal insulin and add mealtime insulin in two or three months.
- Your doctor may want you to start with pre-mixed insulin, which covers both basal and mealtime needs.

If you've been checking your blood glucose levels after meals and the levels are too high, you might think that is a clear sign that you need mealtime insulin. This is not necessarily so. High levels of glucose can suffocate the beta cells. These beta cells are still alive, but they aren't putting out much insulin.

If you use basal insulin, this will clear out the toxic levels of glucose. The beta cells may come back to life and be able to produce enough insulin to cover meals. Relieving glucose toxicity also improves insulin sensitivity. So some doctors prefer to start with basal insulin only, clear out the "noise" of the high glucose levels, and then see what's happening after meals. Because of this, we'll start by describing basal insulin plans.

BASAL INSULIN PLANS: THE INSULINS

Right now, you and your doctor will focus on bringing your fasting glucose level down to your goal. Your doctor may set a goal for you of less than 120 mg/dl, 110 mg/dl, or 100 mg/dl. Your doctor will start you on NPH, glargine, or detemir.

NPH

NPH has been around for years. It's used for basal coverage but it is not a true basal insulin because it has a peak.

You'd likely start with one shot of NPH at bedtime. NPH lasts only 10–16 hours, so if you need 24-hour basal coverage, you'll need to take NPH twice a day.

The absorption of NPH—and therefore its action profile—can vary from day to day. The time of the peak can vary from 4 to 12 hours. Sometimes, the peak works to your advantage. Blood glucose levels naturally rise in the hours before breakfast. This is called the dawn effect. When you take NPH at bedtime, if the peak hits 6–8 hours later, it will coincide with the dawn effect. But if your bedtime is quite early or the NPH peaks earlier in the night (remember that variable absorption), then you may have a nighttime "low" (hypoglycemia).

Pro	Con
• Some insurance plans will cover NPH but not the newer (and more expensive) insulins. Check your coverage.	• More nighttime hypoglycemia (low blood glucose) with NPH than with glargine or detemir. See p. 146.
• When you need mealtime insulin, you can mix NPH with rapid-acting or regular insulin in the same syringe.	• If you do shift work or often travel between time zones, NPH is not the best insulin for you.
• You can fill syringes with NPH ahead of time.	• Variable absorption means unpredictable action curves.
	• NPH is a cloudy insulin. You need to roll the bottle 10 times and tilt it 10 times before drawing each dose.
	• You may need two shots a day for 24-hour coverage.

Glargine

Glargine (brand name Lantus) has a fairly flat action profile and can last the better part of a day (up to 24 hours). Many health care providers and patients prefer it to NPH.

You want to take glargine at the same time every day. Pick the time when you can be most consistent. This might be first thing in the morning, if you wake up at the same time every day, or right before bed, if your bedtime is always the same.

Pro	Con
• Studies show there is less nighttime hypoglycemia with glargine than with NPH.	• Glargine can't be mixed with other insulins.
• Glargine is a clear insulin and doesn't need to be rolled and tilted before use.	• It's acidic, so you can't fill syringes ahead of time.
• Studies show there is less weight gain with glargine than with NPH.	• Some insurance plans don't cover newer insulins such as glargine.
• Most people take it once a day.	
• Glargine is better if you travel across time zones or do shift work. You simply take it at the same time, no matter what time you go to bed.	

Detemir

Detemir (brand name Levemir) also has a fairly flat action profile. It lasts longer than NPH but not as long as glargine.

Pro	Con
• Less nighttime hypo-glycemia with de-temir than with NPH. • It's a clear insulin; does not need to be rolled and tilted be-fore use.	• Can't be mixed in the same syringe with mealtime insulins. • May need to take two shots of detemir a day. • Some insurance plans don't cover newer insulins such as detemir.

BASAL INSULIN PLANS: HOW TO START

Starting Dose

The typical starting dose for basal insulin is 10 units. This is too low for most people. Doctors often start with a low dose to keep from overshooting the goal in the few people who are still sensitive to insulin.

Your doctor may have you start with more than 10 units if you are very heavy. For example, the recommended starting dose of detemir is 10 units or 0.1 to 0.2 units per kilogram of body weight. There are 2.2 pounds per kilogram. A person weighing 330 pounds might start with 15 units or up to 30 units.

In one study, the starting dose of basal insulin was based on the highest fasting glucose level over the previous seven days, measured in millimoles. To convert to millimoles, take blood glucose in mg/dl and multiply by .055. So a person whose highest fasting glucose is 270 mg/dl might start with 15 units $(270 \times 0.055 = 15)$.

Adjusting the Dose

There are several plans for increasing the dose until your fasting glucose is at your goal, a process called titration. All of these plans get you to the same place in about the same amount of time.

Once a Week

In the Treat-to-Target Trial, people started with 10 units of glargine or bedtime NPH and adjusted once a week according to this schedule:

Average of Fasting Glucose for Previous Two Days (mg/dl)	Add _____ Units to Your Dose
180 or higher	+8
140–180	+6
120–140	+4
100–120	+2
less than 100	This was the goal.

Exceptions

- If you have a blood glucose of less than 72 mg/dl (confirmed by a blood glucose meter reading) at any time in the preceding week:
  ☐ Do not increase your dose.

- If you have severe hypoglycemia (so severe that you needed help from someone else) or a blood glucose of less than 56 mg/dl (confirmed by a meter):
  ☐ Cut your dose by 2–4 units.

After two to four weeks, your blood glucose levels will probably be out of the high ranges, and you'll be adjusting by 2–4 units a week. By eight weeks, your fasting blood glucose levels will probably be less than 120 mg/dl.

Two Every Three

With this plan, if your fasting blood glucose level is above goal for three days in a row, you add 2 units to your dose.

One a Day

If you don't like to wait until the next "change day" when your glucose level is obviously too high, your doctor may have you increase your dose by 1 unit every day until you get to your goal.

Slowly but Surely

Don't get discouraged if your fasting glucose doesn't change much in the first few weeks. This is normal. In the Treat-to-Target Trial, it took an average of 10 weeks for fasting glucose levels to approach goal levels.

If you're using NPH, as you get closer to your fasting goal, occasionally check your blood glucose at 2 a.m. to 3 a.m. to see if the peak of the NPH is making you go too low. See Nighttime Lows, p. 146.

SUBJECT: HOW LONG?

FROM: fal

Just curious . . . for any of you who have switched over to insulin from oral meds, how long did it take to get the insulin adjusted to the right dosage? I've been working w/ my endo, faxing in readings once a week, making adjustments. I'm not worried at this point as the adjustments are helping. I'm just interested in how long it's taken others.

FROM: tia

When I started on insulin, it took nearly three months to get things fairly well adjusted. That also included starting on NPH insulin, adding Regular to that for a short time, and finally (I'd asked about it in the beginning) switching to Lantus and NovoLog insulins, which work well for me. I also still take Glucovance (metformin & glyburide) oral meds. I'm glad you're faxing in readings once a week—I think that would have helped me as well! My regular Dr. also left the area shortly after I started on insulin, which didn't help matters. That all being said, insulin is not a drug that you get adjusted once and leave it alone—it's a constant "tweak" for most people.

SUBJECT: FRUSTRATED!

FROM: Nne16

I was started on insulin about a week ago. The Dr said to take insulin w/ evening meal & only take it in AM if FBG was over 126. Since I've been taking the dosage she suggested, I've had to take a dose in AM too because my FBG has yet to be as low as 126.

I know changing to different meds isn't going to make a difference overnight, but I'm not seeing much difference at all from when I was taking Amaryl! My follow-up appt w/ Dr isn't for another week, and at this point I don't have any improvement or anything good to report to her, in spite of monitoring my carb intake to the point of NOT wanting to eat. Yesterday my FBG was over 126, so I took AM dose of insulin then had my 35 carb gram breakfast. Two hours later, my BG level was still too high (ABOVE the 180 recommended).

Am I frustrated? Is it depressing? Am I wondering why bother? A resounding YES to all of those!!

FROM: dec

I hear your frustration. It took me several months to find the right levels of insulin FOR ME. It's like living constantly in a math word problem. You know, if carbs = 30 and starting BS is 120 and exercise at 3 miles per hour for 30 minutes = How many units of insulin!!!

Eventually my endo/staff told me that I could start tweaking the number of units myself based on experience. So with the Lantus, I'd start upping the units by +2 for 4–5 days and watched how that went. If that didn't do it, then I'd increase by +2 for another 4–5 days and observe the numbers. Started at 30 units, and now satisfied at 42 units per night.

Same for the Humalog. I don't want to recommend changing your doses without talking to the doc, but next visit you might ask how you can become your own scientist yourself, so that you can find your own personal best routine. Good luck to you and hang in there.

FROM: tia

I agree. It takes time, and it's nice if you & your Dr. are comfortable with you adjusting your insulin gradually and testing lots as well. Insulin therapy is NOT an exact science . . . but it does work!

Your Final Dose

Do you want to predict what your final dose will be? It's typically 0.3–0.4 units per kilogram of body weight per day (U/kg/day). Remember that there are 2.2 pounds to 1 kg, so you'll have to convert your weight to make these calculations (divide your weight in pounds by 2.2). Your health care provider can do this calculation for you.

- Leaner people may need only 0.2 U/kg/day.
- People who are very overweight (more insulin resistant) may need 0.5 U/kg/day.

So a person who weighs 165 pounds may need 15 units per day ($165 \div 2.2 \times 0.2 = 15$). Someone who weighs 330 pounds may need 75 units per day ($330 \div 2.2 \times 0.5 = 75$).

Your final dose also depends on how many other diabetes medications you take. In the Treat-to-Target study, people were on one or two types of oral agents (diabetes pills). The average final dose was 0.48 U/kg/day. In another study, people were taking two oral agents and needed 0.33 U/kg/day. In a study in which people were taking only one oral agent, the average final dose was 0.69 U/kg/day. So a person who weighs 220 pounds and takes two oral agents may need anywhere from 33 to 48 units per day of basal insulin.

If you take larger doses of insulin, you may be instructed by your health care provider to split it up. If you need more than 50 units per dose, you may be advised to take the second half at a different site or to take half the dose in the morning and half before bed.

SUBJECT: ONCE OR TWICE A DAY?

FROM: S2

My father-in-law was recently placed on Lantus. His doctor recommended that he take 10 units in the morning and 30 units in the evening. Because Lantus is slow acting, this amount did not seem proper, especially since there were to be two injections per day. I was of the belief that Lantus was only used once per day. The doctor became very angry when I questioned him about this. Any suggestions? Thanks.

FROM: cb

There is a wide variety of ways to administer insulin. I take 42 units at night. The doc may have suggested 10 units in the AM to maintain a more level dosage in the bloodstream throughout the day. I've heard of some people who split their Lantus in half, taking half in AM and half in PM. I know that in the evening I seem to hang on to higher BS due to dinner carbs, and I believe that this is due to the previous night's Lantus wearing off. I hadn't thought of what y'all's doctor suggested, and I might give it a try myself. HOWEVER, I would NEVER tolerate a doctor who bristled at ANY question I had about his recommendations. Remember you pay him, not the other way around.

FROM: raz

I have been on Lantus for about two years. I was really struggling with the other insulins. My doctor suggested I try Lantus. It took some experimentation with the dosage, and I have settled on 26 units at night and 15 units in the morning. I have been told that this is an unusual dosage, but it works for me and doesn't seem like such a burden due to the interval between injections. I found that if I used more than 26 units at night my glucose levels would sometimes dip too low. I am also taking Glucophage twice a day. My A1C levels are always in the mid-six range. Don't be afraid to experiment with the dosage (with your doc's okay, of course) a little at a time until you find the right dosage for your lifestyle and metabolism.

"MY FASTING BLOOD GLUCOSE IS AT GOAL. NOW WHAT?"

If you've been using basal insulin for two to three months, you're due for another A1C test. In the Treat-to-Target Trial, almost 60% of people reached the goal of an A1C less than 7% with just basal insulin. Among the people who had A1Cs of 8.5% or less at the start of the study, 75% reached an A1C of less than 7%.

If your A1C is less than 7%:
- Continue with your current diabetes plan.
- Ask your diabetes educator or doctor how often you need to check your daytime blood glucose levels. This depends on your willingness and how much your blood glucose levels change day to day.

If your A1C is greater than 7%, your blood glucose levels are going high during the day.
- Keep checking your fasting glucose levels.
- Also check at other times during the day. Aim for three or more checks a week, rotating the times. For example, one day, check before lunch; the next day, check before dinner; and a third day, check two hours after dinner.
- Write down the results in your blood glucose log.

If the daytime blood glucose levels that you're checking are within goal but your A1C is above 7%, you haven't found the highs yet.
- Check one to two hours after the start of each meal for several days.
- If this doesn't uncover the highs, talk to your diabetes educator.

Blood glucose goals are:
- before meals: 90–130 mg/dl
- 1–2 hours after the start of a meal: less than 180 mg/dl

5

Covering Meals

If you didn't have diabetes, your pancreas would produce extra insulin for two to three hours after a meal. You can mimic that by taking an insulin that has a peak. You need mealtime (bolus) insulin if:

You're on a basal insulin. Your fasting blood glucose level is at your goal, but your A1C is above your goal. This means your blood glucose levels are going too high after one or more meals (see p. 79). Insulin options that your doctor might consider include:

- Adding a rapid-acting (or regular) insulin before one or more meals.
- Switching to a mixed insulin (either premixed or home-mixed).

You haven't started taking insulin yet. Your A1C is over 8.5% or your after-meal blood glucose levels

*are often above 180 mg/dl. Your doctor may decide
to tackle both basal and mealtime insulin needs at
the same time with:*

• Mixed insulin.

*Your A1C is over 7%, and you can't stand the
thought of shots. Your doctor may think about
putting you on:*

• Inhaled insulin, which covers meals (see p. 56).

As you and your doctor decide, here are some
issues to consider.

Which insulins will your insurance plan cover?

• Some plans don't cover the newer insulins.

*Is your lifestyle the same day to day? Do you get up
at the same time? Do you eat about the same
amount of food at about the same time every day?*

• If yes, a plan of twice-a-day premixed insulin
  might be fine.

*Is your life unstructured? Do you have only coffee
on some mornings and big breakfasts other days?
Do you want to be able to have lunch one day at
noon and the next at 2 p.m.? Do you want to sleep
in on your days off?*

• A basal-bolus plan (see p. 89) fits a flexible
  lifestyle better.

Is getting your blood glucose levels to your goal range a high priority for you?

- Basal-bolus plans generally result in better blood glucose control.

Your Diabetes Pills

The sulfonylureas (glyburide, glipizide, etc.) and the meglitinides (Starlix or Prandin) work by getting your pancreas to produce more insulin. If your blood glucose levels are going high after meals even when you're taking enough basal insulin, your pancreas is making very little insulin, and even top doses of those diabetes pills won't help. Your doctor will probably have you stop taking them.

However, your doctor will probably keep you on metformin and possibly a glitazone.

An Option Other than Mealtime Insulin

If your glucose levels go too high after meals, your doctor might consider prescribing exenatide (brand name Byetta). This medication is injected. It is not insulin. You take it before breakfast and dinner. Currently, exenatide is approved for use with sulfonylureas and/or metformin. Some doctors think using basal insulin and exenatide may work well for some people.

SUBJECT: ANYONE USING INSULIN AND BYETTA?

FROM: gj19

I have been on insulin for three years. My lifestyle has changed: 1,700–2,000 calories a day seem to fill me totally. Calorie intake prior to diabetes was 4,000–5,000 a day. I have lost 40 pounds in five months by using strict portion control and exercise. I have noticed that the weight is coming off slower now, and I have much more to lose. Is anybody on insulin and Byetta? I take 70/30.

FROM: BA

I think that Byetta is a very new drug and most people's experience with it so far is alone or in combination with metformin and/or a sulfonylurea, as the manufacturer suggests. Not many people (I'm guessing) are combining it with insulin. That is probably why you haven't gotten more responses from people who can tell you about their experiences. Not that no one is interested—just that you're contemplating a road less traveled. Do let us know what your doctor says. Inquiring minds want to know!

FROM: Dvd

Not sure about how it is going to work for you, but I was put on Byetta yesterday and still have the regular insulin. I don't take insulin unless I am over 150 before a meal though, no regular dose, just sliding scale. My doc told me not to use insulin for breakfast and supper when I take the Byetta and see how that goes. So far I haven't needed the insulin yet and suspect I won't need it with the numbers I am getting so far from the Byetta, which is cool with me cause the lows suck. I will only be using insulin at lunch or bedtime if I am high, but I really don't want to use that evening dose unless it is absolutely needed. Going low at night while sleeping gives me one heck of a hangover the next day, at least I am assuming that is what happens when I feel like that. If I find I still need the insulin I am going to ask for a fast-acting that doesn't have as long a duration as the regular.

ADDING A MEALTIME INSULIN

Let's say you're on a basal insulin and you find you also need mealtime coverage. You can take rapid-acting or regular insulin before meals. If your after-dinner/before-bed blood glucose level is too high, you need mealtime (bolus) insulin at dinner. This is the case for many people, because in the U.S., the evening meal is usually the largest of the day. As your diabetes progresses, you'll need to take bolus insulin before each meal.

- Your doctor might start you with 3–6 units, depending on how high your after-meal glucose level usually is, and adjust up once a week based on your home monitoring results.

- If you are using glargine or detemir, your mealtime insulin will have to be a separate injection. Glargine and detemir can't be mixed with other insulins.

- If you're using NPH, you can mix your meal-time insulin and NPH in the same syringe. See p. 210.

Rapid or Regular: Which Is Better?

Rapid-acting insulins more closely mimic natural insulin release. This is important if your body is making very little insulin.

Think of people hiking up a mountain. Healthy people can start at the bottom and climb all the way to the top with no help. Less robust people may need to drive part of the way up and park. Then they can walk the rest of the way. When they grow older, they'll need to drive all the way to the top.

The blood glucose spike after a meal is like a mountain. People who don't have diabetes produce all the insulin they need and can make it to the top on their own. People who have type 1 diabetes have to be driven all the way up the mountain. They make no insulin on their own, and injected insulin has to do all the work. Rapid-acting insulins, with their sharp peaks, are favored.

Type 2 diabetes falls somewhere in the middle. If you have just crossed over into needing injected insulin, you still make some insulin of your own. Injected insulin doesn't need to do all of the work. It may just need to get you part of the way up the mountain. Then your pancreas may be able to get you the rest of the way up or at least fairly close. You may do fine with regular insulin. You may even be able to manage with NPH.

But as you get older and your diabetes progresses, you'll need a lift that gets you closer to the top. You could take more regular insulin, but as you increase the dose, the duration is longer. You'll still have insulin working after the glucose from your meal is gone, which means your risk of hypoglycemia goes up. So as your diabetes progresses, rapid-acting insulin will probably work better for you.

Regular vs. Rapid-Acting Insulin

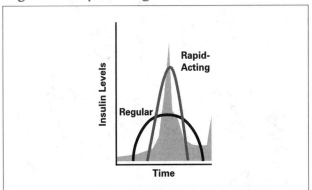

Rapid-acting insulin more closely mimics natural insulin release.

Pro	Con
Rapid-Acting *(aspart, glulisine, lispro)*	
• Less hypoglycemia after meals.	• More expensive than regular insulin.
• More consistent action than regular insulin.	
• Taken right before you eat. More convenient than regular insulin.	
Regular	
• May be better if you have gastroparesis.	• More hypoglycemia several hours after a meal than with rapid-acting insulin.
• May be better for high-fat meals, which lead to later, broader glucose spikes.	• To get the best coverage, you need to inject 30 minutes before you eat. This is often inconvenient.

Caution: Don't Mix Up Your Insulins

You'll now be using two insulins at very different doses. As you get used to the insulin routine, you might start to multitask and do your injection when you're distracted. There have been cases of people taking large doses of rapid-acting insulin when they meant to take their basal insulin. Think of ways to lessen the chance that you will mix up your insulins. Here are some tips.

- Use an insulin pen for one of your insulins and a vial and syringe for the other.
- If you're using vials for both types of insulin, mark all the vials of the rapid-acting insulin with a black X.
- Store your smaller syringes with your mealtime insulin and your larger syringes with your basal insulin.
- If you don't refrigerate your in-use basal insulin, you could keep it in your bedroom and keep your mealtime insulin in the kitchen.

Basal-Bolus Plans

When you take a basal insulin and rapid-acting before each meal, it's called a basal-bolus plan or multiple daily injections (MDI). Basal-bolus plans are sometimes called flexible insulin plans because you don't have to eat on a set schedule. You can eat a big or small meal and take more or less bolus insulin accordingly. You can eat dinner at 5 p.m. one day and 7 p.m. the next.

Multiple Daily Injections (MDI)

When you take a basal insulin plus rapid-acting insulin before each meal, it's called a basal-bolus plan or multiple daily injections (MDI).

Insulin Pumps

You can also deliver a basal-bolus plan using an insulin pump. A pump is a computerized device the size of a pager that holds a two- to three-day supply of rapid-acting insulin. You insert a catheter (a thin, short plastic tube) under your skin, usually at the abdomen, changing to a new site every two to three days. The pump is set to deliver a low level of insulin all day long to cover your basal needs. You program the pump to deliver extra insulin before each meal. The pump can't decide how much insulin you need or when you need it—you still have to test your blood glucose levels and make the decisions.

Pumps cost $5,000 to $6,000, and pump supplies cost about $1,500 a year. With a doctor's prescription, some insurance plans cover some or all of the cost. Medicare also covers insulin pumps for people with type 2 diabetes who meet certain eligibility criteria (benefit category: Durable Medical Equipment).

Get the Best Blood Glucose Control

- Check your blood glucose levels before each meal and at bedtime.
- Adjust your mealtime doses based on your blood glucose level and how much carbohydrate you plan to eat. (See Sliding Scales, p. 127, and Carbohydrate Counting, p. 111.)
- Adjust your doses using pattern management (p. 134).

SUBJECT: BASAL-BOLUS PLANS

FROM: MM4

At first I started with Lantus (one injection a day, no peaks) and continued my oral medications. It was really pretty easy to jab myself with that little tiny needle since it didn't hurt. A little weird at first, but really easy to do. While my fasting sugars got under control, the rest of my day was still looking pretty ugly. So I asked to be put on a rapid-acting insulin (you take that just before a meal). And guess what, two years after I started, I take insulin four times a day (3 rapid + 1 basal), check my sugars three to four times a day, and have an A1C in the low fives. In fact, my A1C hasn't been above 5.4% in two years. My doctor now teases me about my great reluctance to try insulin.

FROM: dec

Started on insulin four years after Dx. Meds had quit being effective, as evidenced by the increase in my A1C from 7.1 (steady for several tests) to 8.6. I sure didn't volunteer for insulin, but soon realized that it was no biggie.

It took a little while to get the drill right, and that included changing types of insulin (NPH and Humulin R, why did he even suggest that?) to the standard routine of Lantus and Humalog.

Insulin seems MUCH more flexible in giving me good control. I was never very good with eating the same amount every day at the same times.

SUBJECT: INSULIN PUMPS

FROM: CN

I am a type 2 diabetic who is pumping. My insurance company covered the costs of my pump. I think it's like automobiles, they all perform the same function, some just have different bells and whistles, but they all get you there. I was on Lantus and Humalog prior to starting the pump.

There are pros and cons to pumping. It is easier to bolus for a snack or meal, but you also have a constant reminder of your disease clinging to your side. I feel it gives me better control and that is my bottom line. I disconnect during my showers (I don't want to think about where to clip it while in the shower—OUCH). I am also an avid fisherman and disconnect while wading so it doesn't get wet. Because I am so active while fishing, my insulin production is sufficient to keep my glucose level under control.

FROM: df7

I've had one for a little over a year and love it. I'm not an electronics wiz but the pump is relatively simple. I went to a two-hour class at my endo's office and was pretty confused and nervous when I left but I got used to it. I called her when I had a question and she would walk me through or answer anything. Also the pump manufacturer has a wonderful support team and can answer any "stupid" question. Luckily I have very good insurance and my pump and supplies cost me nothing—no co-pay or anything. They automatically send me my supplies every three months.

I wish I could say I have "tight control" but I don't. I still have some readings in the low 200s and sometimes my FBS levels are high. As far as inserting the cannula, I use a quick-set device to insert.

The needle does look scary at first. I was plenty nervous the first time but now there's nothing to it. I have to change my site every two days. Now I can do it even half asleep or anywhere.

I disconnect when I shower since that's not a long time, but if I'm going in the pool and know it will be for a while, I "suspend" my pump. That saves a little insulin, as usually I am in the pool or on the deck for a couple of hours. I check my BS and then resume the pump and bolus if I need to. I would say it is definitely much better.

FROM: CN

The first couple of times I inserted a catheter were like the first couple of shots I gave myself, kind of tenuous at first, but you tell yourself "suck it up and get it done." There's an inserter that you pull back and press a button, and it's over with. It is just convincing yourself to press the button. I am currently using a catheter that I manually insert and don't have any problems with the minor "stick."

One of the first things you have to learn with a pump is how much insulin to take to compensate for carbs. My insulin-to-carb ratio is 1 unit for every 10 grams of carbohydrate (you will see people post an I:C ratio of 1:10). Once you discover that, it is programmed into the pump and when you eat, you tell your pump what your current blood glucose level is and how many carbs you will be eating. From that information, it recommends an amount of insulin to take. You are not locked into this amount, though, and you can increase or decrease it. I know that certain foods affect me differently and require more or less insulin and some require that the insulin be administered over a couple of hours (pizza is a killer). All of that can be programmed into the pump so that you do not have to give additional shots.

My basal during the daytime is less than at night because I am more active and do not require as much. When doing yard work or fishing, I can reduce the basal rate for a couple of hours or even disconnect because I have discovered that being very active greatly reduces my insulin requirement. During the winter, I require a higher basal rate than the summer due to reduced activity (the fish don't bite as well, darn it).

Again, you know your body best and how it responds to certain things, you take ownership of this disease and make the adjustments to keep tight control. Hope this answers some of your questions, let me know if there is anything else I can do to enlighten you.

USING MIXED INSULINS

One Shot, Two Jobs

You can get one injection to provide both basal and bolus insulin by using a mixed insulin. You can use either a premixed insulin or mix NPH and mealtime insulin yourself.

Some health care professionals and people with diabetes feel that mixing your own insulins is a hassle. Why bother when you can use a premix? Several are available, with different ratios of basal and bolus insulin. All are available in insulin pens (see p. 194) if you don't want to draw up the dose from a vial.

Other people say that home-mixing is the way to go because it allows flexibility and better control.

Still others say that any plan that uses any mixed insulin is inferior to a basal-bolus plan. They feel that injections are nearly painless, so taking basal and mealtime insulins as separate shots is not a big deal.

	Pro	Con
Home-mixing *You can mix a set dose of NPH with a dose of rapid-acting or regular insulin that can vary with the size of the meal. See p. 210 for instructions.*	• You can change the dose of one insulin without changing the other. • You can use a sliding scale (see p. 127) to get better control.	• Syringes can't be reused.
Premixed *(70/30, 75/25, 50/50)* *See table on p. 51.*	• Premixes are easier to use. • If you have arthritis or poor eyesight that makes home-mixing difficult, a premixed insulin might have the advantage.	• You can't change the ratio of the insulins. • For many people, the trade-off for the convenience of premixed insulin is higher A1Cs and unacceptable hypoglycemia.

Mixed-Insulin Plans

If you aren't on insulin yet, your doctor might start you with one injection of premixed insulin at dinner. The rapid-acting or regular part of the premix covers dinner, and the intermediate-acting portion gives you basal coverage during the night.

If you're already on NPH, your doctor might have you add rapid-acting or regular insulin before dinner. If you normally take your NPH before dinner, you can mix the insulins in the same syringe. If you've found that taking NPH at bedtime works better for you, then you'd give yourself a separate shot of rapid-acting or regular before dinner and NPH at bedtime. Your doctor might have you start with 3 to 6 units and then adjust the dose according to your blood glucose results.

If the mix contains regular insulin, you take the injection 30–45 minutes before the meal (see p. 53, Timing of Regular Insulin). If the mix contains rapid-acting insulin, you take it within 15 minutes of the start of your meal.

When you take mixed insulin twice a day—before breakfast and before dinner—it's called a split-mixed plan. (This is not the same thing as when your doctor instructs you to take some of your basal insulin in the morning and some at bedtime.)

How a Split-Mixed Plan Works

BEFORE-BREAKFAST INJECTION

- The rapid-acting (or regular) portion covers breakfast.
- The delayed-action portion of a premix will give you some coverage at lunch, but not the sharp peak you need if you make very little insulin of your own and eat a decent-sized lunch.
- In a home-mix, the intent is for the peak of the NPH to cover lunch. But the peak is so broad and so variable that it gives poor coverage at lunchtime, and it sometimes leads to late morning or afternoon hypoglycemia. This, in turn, can lead to overeating and weight gain.

BEFORE-DINNER INJECTION

- The rapid-acting (or regular) portion covers dinner.
- The delayed-action or NPH portion provides basal coverage through the night.

Split-Mixed Plan

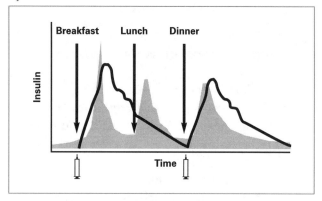

When you take mixed insulin before breakfast and before dinner, it's called a split-mixed plan.

A split-mixed plan doesn't allow for much flexibility. If you're using a premix, you're tied to breakfasts and dinners of set portion sizes. If you eat a larger dinner and try to cover it by taking more premixed insulin before dinner, you'll have too much basal insulin that night.

In a home-mix, the NPH insulin you take before breakfast is going to peak around lunchtime, so you can't skip lunch. If your lunch is delayed, you may have to eat a snack to keep from going low.

A split-mixed plan may work for you if your pancreas is still making a little insulin. But if you've had type 2 diabetes for many years, you'll likely do better with a basal-bolus plan.

A Comparison of Split-Mixed and Basal-Bolus Insulin Plans

Insulin Plan	Pro	Con
Split-Mixed	• Two injections a day.	• Not flexible. • NPH may lead to hypoglycemia mid-morning, mid-afternoon, and at night. • High fasting glucose levels.
Flexible, Basal-Bolus (MDI)	• Flexible. • Better blood glucose control. • Less hypoglycemia.	• Three or four injections.

Premixed Plans: Starting and Adjusting

Your doctor will choose a starting dose based on your weight, which oral agents you're taking, and your blood glucose levels. If you're switching from a basal insulin, the dose will be based on the dose of basal you're taking now.

Recent studies have looked at the best ways to use premixed insulins. In one study of premixed insulin given twice a day, the researchers started with 0.2 U/kg/day for people who were taking metformin and 0.3 U/kg/day for people who were not taking metformin. So a person weighing 220 pounds and taking metformin would start with a dose of 20 units a day ($220 \div 2.2 \times 0.2 = 20$): 10 units before breakfast and 10 units before dinner.

In another study, all of the subjects were taking metformin. Some were also taking a glitazone. Those whose fasting glucose level was less than 180 mg/dl started with 10 units premixed insulin (5 units before breakfast and 5 units before dinner), whereas people with a higher fasting glucose started with 12 units a day (6 units before breakfast and 6 units before dinner). Here is the adjustment plan that was used and the corresponding tables for adjusting doses. Don't follow these without checking with your doctor; he or she may give you a different plan.

One Way to Start Premix Insulin

Starting Dose: 5 or 6 units of 70/30 aspart twice a day

Goal: Fasting and before dinner: 80–110 mg/dl

Adjust: Weekly

Step 1

Check your blood glucose level before breakfast (fasting glucose) and before dinner. Keep track of the results.

Step 2

At the end of the week, look at the numbers for the last three days. If two (or three) of the three values are higher than your target, take the lowest of those values and adjust the dose of insulin that was active at that time according to the charts on p. 104.

- If your fasting glucose is too high, adjust before-dinner insulin.
- If your before-dinner glucose is too high, adjust before-breakfast insulin.
- Call your doctor or diabetes educator if you're not sure what to do. Have your blood glucose log ready.

Check **Fasting Glucose** (Before Breakfast).	
If Two of Last Three Values Are Too High, Look at Lowest. If It Is:	Change **Before-Dinner** Insulin Dose by _____ Units.
180 or higher	+6
141–180 mg/dl	+4
111–140 mg/dl	+2
80–110 mg/dl	no change
less than 80 mg/dl	–2 (decrease dose)

Check Glucose Level **Before Dinner.**	
If Two of Last Three Values Are Too High, Look at Lowest. If It Is:	Change **Before-Breakfast** Insulin Dose by _____ Units.
180 or higher	+6
141–180 mg/dl	+4
111–140 mg/dl	+2
80–110 mg/dl	no change
less than 80 mg/dl	–2 (decrease dose)

Another Way to Start Premix Insulin

Another approach to starting insulin was tested in the 1-2-3 Study.

- People started with 12 units premixed 70/30 aspart before dinner. The dose was adjusted to get the fasting glucose to 80–110 mg/dl.
- After 16 weeks, if A1C was not to the goal of less than 6.5%, the person added a before-breakfast shot of 6 units 70/30 aspart. That dose was adjusted until before-dinner glucose levels were 80–110 mg/dl.
- After 16 weeks, if the person's A1C was still not less than 6.5%, a shot of 3 units 70/30 aspart was added before lunch. That dose was adjusted until the glucose level 2 hours after lunch was 100–140 mg/dl.

Many people were able to reach the A1C goal.

- With one shot a day, 41% had an A1C less than 7%.
- With two shots a day, 70% had an A1C less than 7%.
- With three shots, 77% had an A1C less than 7%.

FROM: sh2

I have been taking insulin for about a month: Lantus (16 units) and a fast-acting before meals (Apidra, 3–5 units). Well to say the least, four shots a day gets to be a pain (no pun intended). I have read on this board about insulin mixes. I guess that means a shot of insulin that includes long lasting and fast? I wanted to talk to my doc, but I kinda would like to know more about it. Does anyone have any advice on this?

FROM: D3

I liked the convenience of the mixed insulin, but I could not make it work for me. I ended up going too high or too low too often.

I was on 70/30 Novolin, which is an NPH and Reg mix. Problem was that no matter what the Dr did, I could not get things just right. Fasting BS was still a bit too high, so he raised my insulin dosage both in the AM and the PM. Then I started going hypo, so he lowered the AM dose. Hypos continued, so he lowered the PM dose. BS then goes back up. Plus, I had a sliding scale insulin to cover when my BS went over 150.

The main problem with a mix is that when you raise or lower the dose, you raise or lower the dose of BOTH insulins, even if only one needs to be changed.

Solution: New endo nixed the mix and put me on NPH and Reg insulin and adjusted the dose of the two insulins. For the NPH, she put me on 25 U in the AM and 22 U in the PM. For the Reg insulin she dosed me by sliding scale. My AM scale was higher than my PM scale. The only adjustments I have made since the change was to increase my PM dose of NPH to 25 U. Since then, I have stayed within the parameters set, not going hypo and, if I do not overeat, not going hyperglycemic either.

Oh and with the mix and the sliding scale, I was still giving myself about three or four injections daily and sometimes more.

If you're tired of MDI (multiple daily injections), maybe it is time to see if you are a candidate for a pump. Mixes do have their place. They are convenient, easy to use, and simple. If you can find the dosage that works for you, then by all means consider it. But you will always have to take at least two injections.

SUBJECT: POOR MAN'S PUMP

FROM: bky

I am considering switching from 70/30 insulin twice a day to the Poor Man's Pump [multiple daily injections/basal-bolus plan] because I am having a problem with control. I tightly control my glucose. A1C typically 5.5 on average (5.3 in March). On non-physically busy days I don't have too many problems, but on very physically busy days I have a lot of lows. So, to "correct" the latter, I don't take my insulin in the AM, which is not a good idea, but beats the readings in the 50s, etc. One of the problems in not taking it in the AM, of course, is that when I eat, I spike higher than I would if I had taken the AM dose. Please share your experience with Poor Man's Pump.

FROM: D3

I was taking 70/30 Novolin and also had a lot of lows, esp. as I got my diet under control and found that I was often eating to feed the insulin or could not exercise because BS was under 100.

My endo says she does not like combos. In her opinion they are easy to use but not easy to dose, meaning you may need more of the NPH but not the rapid-acting or Reg insulin, but with a combo, if you raise one part of the combo, you have to raise both. She does not think you can get tight control with a combo insulin and feels the choice is tight control vs. convenience. I am not sure I believe her 100% because, for some, the combo insulins seem to work, they just did not work for me. I got tired of the lows and then having to feed the insulin to prevent the lows, which hurt my efforts to lose weight.

She separated my insulins, increased my NPH, and put me on a sliding scale for the Reg. So far this has worked. I have not gone hypo but twice since March and that was my fault. First time I was out walking when I peaked, and the second time I was shopping and my lunch was late.

You might do better with separating the insulins you are currently on or switching to MDI with either Lantus/Levemir as your basal insulin and NovoLog or Humalog as your mealtime insulin.

FROM: Tom
When I was on the mix insulins, I had the worst control of my life. I hated everything about the mix. I went on MDI and have much better control. Yes, you have to jab yourself much more than with the mix, but it was worth it. I lowered my A1C down from the 9s and 10s into the low 6s with MDI.

The way I see it, the mix is only good for those people who are scared of insulin and are scared that they are going to kill themselves giving too much fast-acting insulin. Once someone gets the hang of carb counting and injecting, then they should be taken off that and moved to MDI. (IMHO.) I think once you switch to MDI you will feel so much better, and the control will be much better.

Carbohydrate Counting

Meals are made up of various amounts of carbohydrate, fat, and protein. Carbohydrate is the general term for starches and sugars. Carbohydrate is broken down into glucose, which then moves into your bloodstream. This begins within minutes after you eat and continues for several hours.

Carbohydrate raises your blood glucose level. Insulin lowers your blood glucose level. When you balance insulin and carbohydrate, you'll have better blood glucose control. This is called carbohydrate (carb) counting.

How Carb Counting Will Fit into Your Insulin Plan

Basal-only insulin plan: If you're using only basal insulin, you're depending on your pancreas to put out enough insulin after meals. Before you developed diabetes, this was a cinch. Now, it's a bit of a struggle. Carb counting helps you to eat modest amounts of carb at each meal so your body can handle it.

Split-mix plan: If you use premixed insulin, you have a set amount of insulin working after meals. You'll want to eat about the same amount of carb at your meals.

Flexible insulin plan: If you take mealtime insulin and can change the dose, you can add up how much carb you're going to eat and take the amount of insulin that will cover it.

WHERE'S THE CARB?

It's easy enough to talk about carbs and how they affect blood glucose, but it's an entirely different thing to know which foods have carbs and how much per serving.

Foods with notable amounts of carbohydrate

- Grains (rice, oats, flour, pasta, cereal, bread)
- Beans
- Starchy vegetables (potatoes, corn, peas)
- Fruits (fresh, canned, dried, juice)

- Milk products (milk, yogurt)
- Sweets (sugar, hard candy, chocolate, desserts)

Foods with little or no carb (less than 5 g carb per serving)

- Meat, fish, eggs, cheese
- Nonstarchy vegetables (greens, broccoli, eggplant)

People will talk also about carb servings, carb exchanges, or simply "a carb." A carb serving has about 15 grams of carb. Each of these is a carb serving:

- 1 slice of bread
- 1/2 cup cooked cereal
- 1/2 cup corn or 3-inch cob
- 1/2 cup mashed potatoes
- 1/2 cup cooked beans
- 1 small to medium piece of fresh fruit (1/2 of the large fruits you find at your grocer)
- 1/2 cup apple, orange, or grapefruit juice
- 1 cup milk

You can find lists of foods and their carb counts in carb counting and meal planning books. Another great resource is the Nutrition Facts label on packaged food, which lists the grams of carb per serving of that food. You will need to pay close attention to the Serving Size and Total Carbohydrate listed.

Take a look at the food label on p. 115. The information you get from it can help make blood glucose management much easier.

The Total Carbohydrate of 27 grams includes the grams of Dietary Fiber. Fiber is not digested and doesn't raise your blood glucose. Your dietitian might tell you to subtract the grams of fiber from Total Carbohydrate if a serving of the food has 5 or more grams of fiber. In this case, the beverage does not have 5 or more grams of fiber, so you won't have to do any subtraction.

Notice that there is a separate line for Sugars. These are already included in the Total Carbohydrate.

Always make it a point to read the Servings per Container. This juice drink has two servings in its container. One serving has 27 grams of carbohydrate, so if you drink the entire container, then you've consumed 54 grams of carbohydrate.

By reading food labels and finding the information you need on the food you eat, you can begin to easily figure out how much mealtime insulin you will need to take to better manage your blood glucose levels.

Nutrition Facts

Serving Size 8 fl oz (228g)
Servings Per Container 2

Amount Per Serving

Calories 110   **Calories from Fat** 0

	% Daily Value*
Total Fat 0g	**0%**
Saturated Fat 0g	**0%**
Trans Fat 0g	
Cholesterol 0mg	**0%**
Sodium 5mg	**0%**
Total Carbohydrate 27g	**9%**
Dietary Fiber 1g	**5%**
Sugars 25g	
Protein 1g	

*Percent Daily Values are based on a 2,000 calorie diet. Your Daily Values may be higher or lower depending on your calorie needs.

	Calories:	2,000	2,500
Total Fat	Less than	65g	80g
Sat Fat	Less than	20g	25g
Cholesterol	Less than	300mg	300mg
Sodium	Less than	2,400mg	2,400mg
Total Carbohydrate		300g	375g
Dietary Fiber		25g	30g

Calories per gram:
Fat 9   •   Carbohydrate 4   •   Protein 4

FROM: ch12

Ever since my husband has been diagnosed, one month ago, we have really been paying attention to labels. Can anyone explain to me the difference between the number of carbs and "net" carbs? A label will say that it has 20 carbs per serving, but then it says that it only has 4 "net" carbs. We are so confused. Thank you for your help.

FROM: BA

It is a very confusing subject, and even a little controversial. American labels include fiber as part of the total carbohydrates. Fiber is not digestible, does not supply calories, and, most important for our purposes, does not cause the blood sugar to rise. In fact, fiber has the helpful property of slowing down the absorption rate of carbs.

A food that has 21 total grams of carbohydrates, including four grams of fiber, has 17 grams of digestible carbs. Are you with me so far? So on that item, the vendor could claim "17 net carbs." Most of the time most labels don't say this, but it is true nevertheless. Vendors tend to use it when they think it might be a good selling point.

Another type of carbohydrate that isn't digestible in a way the fully impacts blood sugar levels is sugar alcohol (which is neither sugar nor alcohol). For purposes of counting carbs to manage BS, subtract half of the sugar alcohol carbs from the total carbs. If a candy bar has 31 grams of total carbohydrates and 10 of those are from sugar alcohol, its "net carb" count is $31 - 5 = 26$.

Some people count only net carbs. They (we, actually, since this is how I do it) subtract the fiber or half of the sugar alcohol no matter what its amount. Some people only subtract the indigestible carbs if they are over a certain amount, typically 5 grams. Using net carbs is a fairly new concept, and some people don't do it at all—they count all the carbs, even though some of those carbs don't raise BS levels.

Congratulations on paying attention to labels. That is a great start for following a food plan.

FROM: Tou

Yes, it is confusing. However, never lose sight of the real goal: keeping those blood sugar levels down and under control. If what you eat doesn't give you a high blood sugar spike, then it is a fine addition to your diet. On the other hand, if it does, it has to become a no-no, regardless of what the label states. The labels should be your guides, not absolute facts. A year after my Dx, I find that many of the things that initially gave me some real problems are now perfectly fine to include in my meals.

FROM: BA

Two very excellent points. Label reading is important, but meter reading is an even better guide. According to the label and my food plan, I "should" be able to eat oatmeal for breakfast, but my meter tells me otherwise. And my ability to process certain foods or amounts of carbs has seemed to change somewhat as I've lost weight and started exercising and my BS has gone down. So it is good to keep in mind that things change. Label reading and understanding the concept of net carbs is an excellent start.

SUBJECT: WHAT TO DO ABOUT FIBER?

FROM: Mc

My doctor said to take 1 U Humalog for every 10 g of carbs and adjust as needed. When counting carbs, does fiber count or should I subtract it? Should I also count the carbs from low-starch veggies, like broccoli? When "adjusting as needed," should I just go up one dose at a time?

FROM: mk

Sounds like your Dr. is starting you out conservatively, which is good. If you can see a CDE to help learn how to adjust your dosage, you might feel more comfortable with doing both. I choose to count carbs, not subtract fiber and don't count the low-carb veggie carbs at all. This is up to you. A CDE or dietitian could help you with what to do in this area, too.

FLEXIBLE INSULIN PLANS

Let's say you eat salmon with a side of broccoli for dinner. The next night, you have spaghetti and garlic bread. The first dinner is low in carb, and the second is high in carb. If you're on a flexible insulin plan, you would take less mealtime insulin before the low-carb dinner and more before the high-carb dinner. You'd figure your insulin dose based on the grams of carbohydrate in the meal.

People with type 2 diabetes typically need 1 unit of rapid-acting (mealtime) or regular insulin to cover 10 grams of carbohydrate (a 1:10 ratio). If you are very insulin resistant, 1 unit of insulin may cover only 5 grams of carbohydrate.

You don't have to figure this out on your own. Your dietitian or diabetes educator will look at your total insulin dose and your blood glucose records, do some calculations, and estimate your ratio. Blood glucose monitoring before and after a meal will guide your adjustments. You might change the ratio several times over the course of several months before you hit on the best ratio.

SUBJECT: RATIOS

FROM: FT

I know there is supposed to be so many units of insulin to so many carbs. I think it's between 10–15 carbs per unit, depending on the person. I'm going to the bookstore and try to educate myself on insulin. I should have been given better training with insulin. How can they expect anyone to be proficient at something if a person has not been properly trained? Actually, I'm getting pretty annoyed with it. Thank you kindly for your reply. Take care and be well.

FROM: BK

I base my short-acting insulin (NovoLog) on 1 U per 15 grams of carbs, and this seems to work well for me. If I eat after exercising, I might back off a unit or two of insulin because I know that the exercise will help with my postprandial bump as well. I try to have no more than 45 grams of carbs in a meal and 30 for a snack, as that works best for me. And for some metabolically inexplicable reason, eating salad with a meal keeps my glucose levels down.

FROM: al

During the day, say lunch, I take 1 U of Humalog for every 30 g of carbs. At my big meal at night it is 1 U to every 15–20 g, depending on my evening activity.

Your insulin sensitivity may change during the day, so you might use different insulin-to-carb ratios at different times of the day. You might have a different ratio on days that you exercise, because exercise makes you more sensitive to insulin and 1 unit of insulin will cover more carbohydrate.

Blood glucose monitoring will show you what happens when you eat certain foods. For example, high-fat, high-protein meals usually lead to a delayed rise in blood glucose. Pizza is notorious for this.

SUBJECT: TRIAL AND ERROR

FROM: fm

You will find that certain foods digest at different rates and that can affect the insulin's effectiveness. I tend to play it pretty conservative. What I will do is adjust the time I take my Humalog. For myself, if I eat certain foods like a slice of pizza, I inject after my meal. I do the same for pasta because both of those foods peak after the one hour peaking of the Humalog. It is a trial and error thing with me, as I have discovered how my body reacts to certain foods, as well as how the insulin reacts to certain foods. It's all a bit confusing at times.

FINDING A REGISTERED DIETITIAN

You'll want to see a registered dietitian (RD) to get help in starting carb counting and making insulin work for you. Many states also require dietitians to be licensed, so you'll often see that qualified individuals will also have an LD, for licensed dietitian. An RD who is also a certified diabetes educator (CDE) is an excellent addition to your health care team.

To Find a Registered Dietitian

- Check your health plan's list of preferred providers.
- Go to the American Dietetic Association, www.eatright.org. Click on "Find a Nutrition Professional." Two more clicks and you'll get to the search page. Enter your zip code and under "Select a Specialty" click "Diabetes."
- Go to the American Association of Diabetes Educators at www.aadenet.org and click on "Find an Educator." Look for CDE and RD.

If you have Medicare Part B (for services outside of the hospital), then medical nutrition therapy (MNT) is a covered service, but you must go to an RD who is a Medicare provider.

If you have health coverage through your employer, call your health plan and ask if they cover medical nutrition therapy. Ask if you will need a referral from your doctor.

If you don't have any insurance coverage, consider paying for sessions yourself. Some dietitians offer a package that includes a number of sessions. Medical nutrition therapy can keep you healthier over the long term, and this makes the expense well worth it.

SUBJECT: TWO-HOUR READINGS . . . WHY?

FROM: HT7

Can somebody help me understand the reasoning behind the two-hour post-meal reading? I guess I must have fallen asleep when this subject was being discussed, so here goes.

My understanding was that you test before a meal and then two hours after a meal and that there should not be any more than a 40-point difference. Got that part; but here's where I get confused. I thought that meant that the two-hour mark was when you "peaked" and that was why you tested at that point. After meeting with my new CDE (who I love) yesterday, I asked her to explain it again and she did, but I still don't get it. She said that you peak around an hour and that by the two-hour mark, you should be going down. How do you know that you are going down at that point, unless you test at the one-hour AND two-hour marks? Have I totally missed the whole point? I am really confused right now. Any help would be greatly appreciated.

I had exactly the same confusion you are experiencing. We do peak sooner than two hours after eating. I did a lot of testing on myself—20 times on a couple of days—and discovered that I generally peak at 45–60 minutes after meals. By then, we should be well on the way back to our baseline within a couple of hours. The glucose in our blood should be delivered to the muscle and brain cells that need it, and the cells should have enough insulin to be able to take it in. So testing after two hours helps us see whether things are working as they "should" be.

Testing after one hour would help determine what our highest BS levels are. So when we test depends on what we (or our doctors) want to know.

FROM: **BL**

A lot of us do test at the one-hour mark because we found out we were missing harmful spikes. Just last night I got curious (OK, maybe stupid instead of curious) and tried Cracklin' Oat Bran again and tested just after an hour. The results were not pretty. They were the same ugly results as last time I tried it several months ago.

It sounds like you have a good educator. I had to learn about the one-hour thing here. I have built a list of safe foods that don't spike me. Strangely, 12 grams of carbs and 3 grams fiber in large juicy strawberries won't do the same thing as 1/3 cup

Cracklin' Oat Bran (15 grams of carbs and 2 grams of fiber). Strawberries don't bother me at all.

FROM: Nih

Here's what I do. If I've had this particular food before and I know I'm all right with it, then I test two hours after a meal just to reaffirm that I'm on the right track. If it's a new food (or a particular food that for some reason I can't get through my thick skull that I SHOULDN'T eat), I test one hour after eating to see what my peak number is and then also at two hours to see how much my BG has dropped. I've done that twice now with sushi and twice I've peaked at 240 then dropped to 178 after two hours, and yes, it's confirmed, I cannot eat rice.

FROM: lod

I'm not so sure that it matters when you test, nearly so much as that you do test and use that information to improve control. The nice thing about picking one time and sticking to it is that when you look back at numbers in a few days, or a week, to compare them with current numbers, they mean more if you know when they were taken.

FROM: Tlt

About a month ago, I got caught up in the one-hour testing and then I always tested two hours afterwards. I was very focused on the one-hour test—obsessed, actually. I had no reason for it, though, because I rarely peak over 140 at one hour. About 85% of my two-hour readings are below 110 and never over 140. Anyway, I had a meeting with my dietitian to get some more pointers, and we talked about the one-hour test because she saw how obsessed I was with it. She also called in the CDE to discuss this with me.

The result: Forget the one-hour test unless you want to see how a new food affects you. Focus on the two-hour mark. I test at one hour and then two hours if I try a "regular" portion of a new food or a new snack, but those days of one-hour obsession for every meal are over. As it was explained to me, when you peak between 45 minutes to one hour, it is really not a sustained prolonged peak—it's done and over with (hopefully). But a two-hour peak that is high, especially if it is really high, is not what you are aiming for.

Sliding Scales and Pattern Management

CORRECTING THE PAST: SLIDING SCALES

On a flexible insulin plan, you'll check your blood glucose level before each meal. Many times your blood glucose levels won't be in your goal range. This is normal. It's not your fault, it's just life. Perhaps you ate more than you planned or exercised more than usual.

Even if you eat the exact same thing every day and keep your activity level the same, things you can't control will affect your blood glucose levels. For example, how quickly your body absorbs insulin will vary from day to day. This is especially true of NPH insulin. Stress can raise blood glucose. Hormones can affect your glucose levels, too. So expect the unexpected result.

FROM: mm

It's like you do all of the right things, yet your BG has a mind of its own. It's so very, very frustrating!

FROM: LN

I will go through a few high weeks and then a few low weeks without rhyme or reason. I'm not great for writing down everything I eat and how much I exercise, so it is possible that if I did, I might know why that happens, but my suspicion is that nothing much changes in those periods. But I have learned to avoid stressing about it because as an invisible friend says, "What goes up also comes down." And it always does.

FROM: lan

A couple of great things about walking and exercise: the exercise you do now has a ripple effect. It can ripple into tomorrow's glucose readings, too. I was delighted when I heard that from my diabetes educator. That is why our glucose readings are sometimes baffling. They might represent some of what you did yesterday, not just what you ate two hours ago.

When your premeal blood glucose levels are out of range, do you just have to shrug and do nothing? No. On a flexible insulin plan, you can adjust your insulin dose to take care of these normal ups and downs so they don't ripple through the day. You take a little more of your mealtime insulin if your blood glucose is high, a little less if it's low. (You can't do this with a premix, because you'd also be changing the dose of basal insulin.)

You'll need a sliding scale that has been worked out just for you. Your doctor or diabetes educator will factor in your weight, activity level, insulin sensitivity, and other medical conditions. Here is an example (yours may be different).

Sliding Scale for L.B.

When Blood Glucose Before Your Meal Is	Use Carb Counting to Figure Out Your Meal Time Insulin Dose and Then Add or Subtract as Below:
<60	Subtract 2–4 units
61–80	Subtract 1–2 units
81–120	Take usual dose
121–150	Add 1 unit
151–180	Add 2 units
181–210	Add 3 units
For every additional +30	+1 unit

You can also correct for highs and lows by changing when you take your mealtime insulin. If you use a rapid-acting insulin, you usually take your insulin right before you start to eat. When your premeal blood glucose is below 70 mg/dl, your sliding scale may have you delay your shot until after you start eating, in addition to reducing the dose. For the timing of regular insulin, see p. 53.

SUBJECT: CORRECT A HIGH?

FROM: ja8

I am new to insulin. I take 56 units of Lantus at night, and I'm on Apidra when I eat. How much of that I take depends on my numbers and what I'm about to eat. I've been on Apidra for about a week and a half. With a few exceptions, my numbers two hours after eating have been good. I have had two readings of around 222 two hours after eating. My question is if you're on insulin and you get a high number two hours after eating, do you take a little more insulin to try to get your numbers to come down? I know you wouldn't take as much as you would if you were eating. I'm talking like 2 or 3 units, depending on your reading.

Example my dr told to me with the Apidra: I test before I eat. I should take 1 unit for every 35 over 150 then add 8–12 units for the food I'm about to eat. So let's say I test and my reading is 300, that's 150 over 150. Take that 150 divide by 35 which gives you 4 units just to get my sugars down. Then I would add let's say 10 units for the food I'm about to eat. So I would give myself 14 units of Apidra. This formula has worked very well for keeping my numbers down. But it does make sense that after I eat if my numbers are very high then I could give myself a little more insulin to bring them down. I have an appt this week and will ask my dr about this, but I also want to know what you all think.

FROM: lod

If your morning numbers are good, and you FREQUENTLY have high readings at two hours after your meal, then your doctor might decide to increase the amount of insulin you take before meals. Remember, an occasional high number does less damage than a really low one, so especially at the beginning, while you and your doctor are learning how you react to different doses, he or she is probably being a little conservative about the amount of insulin that is being prescribed. You might find there are other things you can do, too, like counting carbs and measuring portion size more carefully or doing a little exercise to help lower that high number.

One problem with adding more insulin between meals is that then the extra insulin will still take some time to go to work and may just be reaching its peak at about the time you start your next meal. That makes it harder to dose accurately for the next meal.

At some point, your doctor may give you more freedom to adjust your own insulin dose, but for now, unless you have a couple of readings in a row over 250 or so, you probably don't need to do anything more. You can just take note and keep track of anything you can think of that might be affecting your numbers. Then you can discuss it with your doctor at your next appointment.

FROM: sh2

Hi. I take 13 units of Lantus at night and 3–7 units of Apidra before meals. I just saw my endo and asked him your very same question. He said taking an extra unit once in a while would not be a problem but not all the time. If you do it too often, you can run into overlapping doses, which you don't want to do on a continual basis. It works for me whenever I probably don't calculate the correct amount of carbs and the BG goes a little high. Good luck, and as always call your doc and ask.

FROM: fm

I just started on Humalog about seven weeks ago, and I'm still tweaking my dosage. If my numbers are high after my meal, I do not give myself more unless they are above my high target range two hours or more after my meal. When I do make a correction, I try to figure on 1 unit per 30 points in blood glucose. Let's say that my three-hour number is 180 and I want to get it down to 120, I would take a 2-unit correction. I have rarely needed to do this. I would call your doctor and ask him or her about correction dosages. I asked mine, so I felt comfortable doing it.

FROM: cf

As far as the after-meal highs, as a general rule, you should not take insulin injections any closer than two hours apart or you greatly increase the possibility of a low. If I am high two hours after a meal, I take more insulin on a custom sliding scale that my doc worked out for me. This scale is substantially different than a premeal sliding scale. I don't take any unless I am over 200 two hours after a meal, and then it is not anywhere near a premeal injection. I start with 1 unit and increase every 50 points, so if I am at 320 at the two-hour mark, I take another 3 units. Ask your doc for more info on this because your chance of a low is greatly increased and most will not suggest a make-up dose until you are still high at your next meal.

SUBJECT: HI READING

FROM: muy
About 45 minutes ago, I took my blood glucose and received a reading saying "HI." I checked my user handbook, and it said that it means over 500. I took Humalog, waited 25 minutes, and retested. It was 138. I checked it again about five minutes ago, and it was 193. What might cause such a HUGE fluctuation? Could it be related to the meter? And what else might be wrong physically?

FROM: QL14
I am going to say that most likely it was meter error. I would suggest testing again immediately if you get a reading that says HI.

FROM: Hos

You should always have a second meter around. It could be dangerous to use that much insulin at once. I never trust a reading if it doesn't make sense. I learned the hard way when I had to stay up and drink sugar water to keep alive.

FROM: hp1

One time I had a similar very high reading that puzzled me until I realized I had eaten a juicy apple and had some juice on my finger when I tested.

FROM: BL62

I had my meter goof up before. It shot up to 500. I freaked and checked my BS again, and my levels were normal. I tried again after, say, 30 minutes, and it was still normal. Sometimes equipment fails. I do have a second one as backup now.

CHANGING THE FUTURE: PATTERN MANAGEMENT

You check your blood glucose before lunch. It's a little high. No problem. You use your sliding scale to correct for it. The next day at lunch, it's a little high again. You use your sliding scale to correct for it. On the third day, you're high again before lunch.

You may start to wonder: "Can't I do something to prevent these out-of-range numbers instead of just reacting to them after the fact?"

Yes, you can. It's called pattern management. A pattern is when your blood glucose is

- high at the same time of day three days in a row
- low at the same time two days in a row

When you see a pattern, the next day you change the insulin that was active at the time of the pattern. You'll change the dose by only 1 or 2 units at a time. You were doing pattern management when you first started using insulin. That's how you got to the dose that controlled your fasting glucose levels.

If you use a premix insulin and want to correct a pattern you see at only one time of day, you'll have to switch to insulins that you mix yourself or to a basal-bolus plan. Then you can adjust the dose of just one of the insulins.

It's not always obvious which insulin is affecting which blood glucose result, so ask your doctor or diabetes educator for instructions. See p. 136 for guidelines.

When This Glucose Reading Is Out of Range Three Days in a Row	Adjust This Insulin
Fasting	Long acting (If you adjust your long-acting insulin, you may need to adjust your rapid-acting insulin as well.)
After breakfast or before lunch	Breakfast insulin
After lunch or before dinner	Lunch insulin
After dinner or bedtime	Dinner insulin

Pattern Management: A To-Do List

- Make sure your meter is accurate.
  - ☐ Check your meter with a control strip.
  - ☐ Ask your diabetes educator to check your technique and to check your results against lab results.
- Check your blood glucose level four times a day.
  - ☐ Before meals and before bed.

- Write down your results in a blood glucose log.
  - You may want to highlight lows in one color and highs in another color, so you can see patterns more easily.

SUBJECT: DO YOU ADJUST YOUR INSULIN DOSES?

FROM: ES

Does anyone here ever adjust their own insulin a few units up or down without permission from their doctor? I mean . . . we are the ones who know how we eat and are checking our blood glucose. I don't mean getting too radical with insulin. Would anyone admit it? Or is it one of those unwritten rules that people do but never talk about?

FROM: mh

I think most people who have been taking insulin for a while have been taught by their doctors how to make some adjustments on their own. In those cases, though, the dosage depends largely on being able to count carbs and then matching insulin to carbs. Better work on the carb counting first.

FROM: AB

Yes, I will do that if I think more or less insulin will stabilize my BS. Example: I started on 10 units of

NovoLet 70/30 and crept up to 20 at 2 units a time until I thought things looked better. I do more testing when I change the units. Then I tell my doctor what I did on my next visit, loaded with Excel graphs to show him the effect. He usually agrees with me, but once he did change my insulin, telling me that Lantus wasn't cutting it and that I needed a second insulin and less Lantus.

FROM: MM4

I've been using insulin for about three years now and yes, I adjust my insulin all of the time, especially the rapid-acting insulin. Can you share what kind of insulin(s) you take? The newer regimens of a basal insulin taken once a day (Lantus) followed by a rapid-acting insulin at mealtime (NovoLog or Humalog) are much different than insulin regimens that use premixes like 70/30. My Lantus dose was adjusted until I got a good series of fasting levels and has pretty much stabilized for the past year or so. My Humalog dose can be adjusted every time I eat (depends on my premeal sugar level and the amount of carbs I eat). It seems to work well, because my A1C has been consistently around 5% for the past two years. I started on Lantus (with my orals too) and graduated to the rapid insulin when I still couldn't get good control. My doctor was going to prescribe 70/30, but I insisted on the rapid acting. He tells me that this is now the standard insulin regimen they use for patients going on insulin. I guess I was the poster boy for this in the practice.

FROM: pv

I have been on insulin for five short months and have been adjusting my dose from the first week. At first, the Dr was surprised but now only asks what I am taking and looks at my numbers. So far, so good. He told me that more people should take such an active role in their treatment. Whatever adjustments you make should be done slowly over the course of a few days and by a few units at a time. You definitely don't want to overdo it and go too low. Everything takes time. Don't push it, and good luck.

8

The "Lows"
Prevention and Treatment

A blood glucose level that is too low is called hypoglycemia. Ask your doctor what blood glucose levels to watch out for. In general, if you're a healthy adult, below 70 mg/dl is considered too low. Your doctor might set the "safe level" higher for you if any of the following apply:

- You have heart problems.
- You are elderly, especially if you live alone.
- You have a job where hypoglycemia would be dangerous.
- You have trouble knowing when your blood glucose is low.

Many things can cause hypoglycemia: too much insulin, too little food, a delayed meal, a meal with too little carbohydrate, more exercise than usual, or alcohol on an empty stomach. Hypoglycemia is more common just before meals, after hard exercise, and when insulin is peaking. Sometimes it occurs at night when you're sleeping.

SUBJECT: EXERCISE AND LOWS

FROM: db2

I am newly using insulin and starting with the 70/30 premix insulin pen. I have gone to the gym and need to figure out when and how to do a workout. My blood sugar dropped to 47 and to 73, and then I get lows in the middle of the night. Not sure if I should just not use the insulin if I am planning on going to the gym. Anyone have experiences or knowledge about this?

FROM: D3

I still tend to go hypo when I exercise, so I avoid exercising when my insulin is peaking and I also make sure that I take Life Savers candies with me. I have found for moderate walking I need to eat one Life Saver every 15–20 min for as long as I am walking. I am still having problems with going hypo, so I am trying to convince the Dr to change me over to an insulin pump. That way I can stop the pump when I am exercising and do not have to worry about the "insulin on board" issues.

FROM: E

I prefer to start exercise about 30–45 minutes after I eat. When you exercise before eating, you can go too low. If you start at about 30 minutes after, you start when that digesting glucose is starting to hit your bloodstream, so it is taken up more quickly.

FROM: Al

I've been a T2 guy for over 30 years now. About 10 years ago, I started on Lantus insulin with 15 units daily, which has now risen to 52 units daily. I take one injection a day in the morning. The only trouble I used to have is that vigorous exercise would bring me to the hypo level and then I would have to quit. I've learned to anticipate the level of my workouts and now adjust my insulin (reduce about 20%) on days I intend to have a more vigorous workout.

During the workouts, I take a blood measurement at various break points. If my glucose level is below 100, I take 30 g of carbs for each projected half hour of further workout. If I get it wrong, I can't go any further, so I just rest and go home.

This proves the value of exercise relative to controlling BS levels. If I ever get to the point of a consistent exercise schedule and a consistent energy consumption rate, I believe I could permanently reduce my insulin level.

SUBJECT: TOOK WRONG INSULIN

FROM: f6

My husband accidentally took 40 units of Humalog instead of 40 units of Lantus. He woke me to tell me that he did this and that he drank a soda and ate some cookies to cover it. Then he went to bed. That was an hour ago, and I am still awake, not knowing what to do. Any suggestions?

FROM: lod

Humalog begins to work in about 15 minutes, peaks between one and two hours, and lasts for about three to four hours. That means that his Humalog is getting near its peak right now.

I think it would be wise to wake him now and get him to check his glucose level right now and every half hour until the Humalog wears off, or do it for him if you can. If his glucose is low, he needs to eat something else sweet and retest every 15 minutes until it returns to a more normal level. Then, he will probably need to take some extra Humalog tomorrow to replace the missing Lantus, until he takes his usual Lantus tomorrow evening.

Another thing you can do is to call your local emergency room or perhaps your insurance company's hotline, if they have one, for professional advice. Certainly call for help if his blood sugar is low and he is too disoriented to cooperate with you in eating something to raise it.

FROM: f6

Thanks for your reply. You've calmed me down already. I woke him just a few minutes ago, and he says he's fine and seems OK. But I am going to make him test his BG just to make me feel better. The most Humalog he ever takes is 10 units, so I wasn't sure if I should panic or not. Apparently not, which is comforting to know.

FROM: lod

Can you tell us how things are going today?

FROM: f6

Good morning, and it is one thanks to your advice. At 4:30 a.m., he was at 61, so thanks to your advice, I knew to give him six ounces of juice. He went back to bed and got up this morning at 151 BG. A little high, but better than those awful crashes. I didn't get a lot of sleep, but I didn't worry nearly as much as I would have without the information provided here. It's good to know that I can deal with situations like this and have them turn out OK. Last night was a real oops!

FROM: SA

He might want to label one of those bottles with a BIG RED marking pen, so it stands out like a sore thumb.

SYMPTOMS

If your blood glucose is going too low, or if it's simply dropping fast, your body releases epinephrine (adrenaline).

Symptoms of Low Blood Glucose

Shaky	Impatient
Nervous	Anxious
Sweaty or clammy	Light-headed
Irritable	Hungry

NIGHTTIME LOWS

Do you find your pajamas and sheets damp in the morning? Have you had restless sleep and nightmares? When you wake up, do you have a headache or still feel tired? You may have had a low during the night.

Check your blood glucose levels around 2 a.m. or 3 a.m. for a couple of days to find out if you're going low at night. If you are, tell your health care team. They'll advise you on how to change your diabetes plan to prevent nighttime lows.

NPH and Nighttime Lows

If you use NPH as your basal insulin, remember that it has a peak that can cause nighttime lows. Here are some ways to avoid this.

- If you're taking NPH before dinner as part of a mixed insulin, switch to separate shots: rapid-acting before the meal and NPH at bedtime (the doses will likely have to be changed).
- Eat a snack before bed. Talk to your dietitian. You don't want to add unneeded calories. You might want to eat less at dinner to allow for a bedtime snack.

■ Switch from NPH to detemir or glargine.
These insulins have a lower risk of nighttime lows.

MISSING THE SIGNS

You may not get or you might miss the early warning signs of hypoglycemia if:

- You have even mild autonomic neuropathy
  (nerve damage from diabetes).
- You have had diabetes for many years.
- You have had a recent bout of hypoglycemia.
  Hypoglycemia makes your body less reactive to
  the next bout. You may not get symptoms until
  your blood glucose drops to even lower levels.
- You're keeping your blood glucose levels
  near the normal range. Your body gets used
  to often being close to 70 mg/dl,
  and it doesn't react as much when you
  dip below that. That's why it's important to
  monitor your blood glucose levels more when
  you aim for near-normal glucose levels.

When you can't recognize the symptoms of low
blood glucose, it's called hypoglycemia unawareness.

Is It Really Low?

You can develop symptoms of hypoglycemia when your blood glucose is falling rapidly but is still above 70 mg/dl. For example, if your blood glucose drops from 180 to 100 rapidly, you might get chills or start sweating.

Check your blood glucose level. If you don't find out for sure whether you're low, you may be treating a "non-low." That can lead to high glucose levels, and weight gain if it happens a lot.

On the other hand, you might brush off symptoms. Early warning signs are easy to miss. Your heart is beating faster. Is it nervousness or low blood glucose? Don't wait to see if the symptoms go away. Only a blood glucose check can tell you for sure.

What if you don't have your glucose monitor when you feel that your blood glucose is going low? Don't wait. When in doubt, always treat.

Over time, you'll gain confidence in your ability to manage your diabetes. You may think you can check your blood glucose less often. Be careful that you don't convince yourself that you can tell your glucose level by how you feel. Research shows that few people can guess their blood glucose level. Guessing is dangerous, particularly if your blood glucose level tends to fall with very little warning.

TREATMENT: TAKE 15, WAIT 15

When you're having a low blood glucose reaction, your body needs glucose fast. You need to eat or drink something with sugar or starch. By now, you probably have your favorite form of "pocket sugar" that you keep with you at all times.

When you first notice a reaction, check your blood glucose level if you can. Then "Take 15, Wait 15." Take about 15 grams of glucose or other fat-free carbohydrate. You want to avoid fat because it slows the absorption of carbohydrate and adds calories that you don't need.

Carb Sources

Each of these has about 15 grams of carbohydrate:

- 2–5 glucose tablets, depending on the brand (this is the best treatment)
- half a can of regular soda
- 1/2 cup (4 oz) of orange juice
- 5–7 Life Savers candy
- 10 gumdrops
- two large lumps of sugar
- one tablespoon of honey or corn syrup
- 1 tube of Cake Mate decorator gel
- 1 cup of skim milk

Recheck your blood glucose after 15 minutes. If your blood glucose hasn't come up enough, take another 15 grams of carbohydrate and retest in 15 minutes.

After you treat the reaction, if it's the middle of the night or if your next meal is more than an hour away, also eat a snack.

The symptoms of hypoglycemia often linger after blood glucose levels are back in the normal range. Resist the urge to eat until you feel better or your blood glucose will likely go too high and you'll have taken in extra calories.

If you have lows regularly—say, once or twice a week—report this to your health care team. You don't want to always be chasing lows and gaining weight because of it. A change in your diabetes plan should be able to prevent the lows.

If you take a sulfonylurea and have a low, your risk of another low remains high for many hours. Call your health care team. You may be told to check your blood glucose levels every two hours for 12–24 hours.

Alpha-glucosidase inhibitors (acarbose or miglitol) don't cause hypoglycemia. However, if you also take a sulfonylurea, meglitinide, or use insulin, hypoglycemia can occur. In these cases, use pure glucose (tablets or gel) to treat the low. Acarbose and miglitol slow the breakdown of many other carbohydrates, so those carbohydrates won't be effective in treating a low blood glucose.

FROM: gg

I ate two small chocolate donuts and drank a glass of chocolate milk. It was the first thing I thought about.

FROM: mj

When you have a low, you should not eat sweets with fat in it such as chocolate. It takes too long to digest. Drink a half a can of real soda, eat about 16 Skittles or 8 jelly beans, or drink a half a glass of orange juice. You can also buy tablets from the pharmacy for this. You should then check your BG in 15 minutes. If it is still low, then drink or eat more.

FROM: gg

OK. I haven't tried the glucose pills yet. I'm kind of scared of another thing to have to carry around. But maybe I will try. Are they expensive?

FROM: k11

Glucose tablets are roughly one to two dollars for a package. I have found them helpful several times when I was shopping or out somewhere and I could tell that I was getting low enough that I felt dizzy and desperately needed food. It's a quick pick up if you get too low. But let me share a caution about the glucose tablets. If you use them to get you out of a low, plan on eating real food within a half hour or so. I have found that they can help, but if I don't eat food soon after taking the glucose tablets, then I will go low again. My mother is the same way.

SEVERE HYPOGLYCEMIA

If the early signs and symptoms of hypoglycemia go unnoticed, you could develop severe hypoglycemia. Your brain will not be getting enough glucose. You'll get so drowsy or confused that even if someone hands you juice, you can't drink it. If they try to force you to drink or eat, you could choke. You can become unconscious or have a convulsion.

Severe hypoglycemia is a real emergency. Someone needs to call 911 or give you a shot of glucagon.

Glucagon is a hormone that makes the liver release stored glucose. This raises the blood glucose level, and the person usually regains consciousness. Glucagon doesn't work in people who have no stores of glucose in the liver, such as alcoholics.

Glucagon is available by prescription. It's injected like insulin. Someone you trust needs to be trained how to fill the special glucagon syringe and how to give you the shot.

You should respond to glucagon in 2–10 minutes. When you are fully awake, you should be offered sips of juice. If you can keep that down, you should be offered food. If you are still confused or unconscious 15 minutes after the glucagon injection, someone should call 911. After the crisis is over, notify your doctor that you had a low that was severe enough that you needed glucagon.

Anyone who uses insulin needs to have glucagon in the house. It stays good for two years after it is manufactured. When it expires, get a new glucagon kit. Then have someone in your family practice mixing up the glucagon in the expired kit.

WEAR A MEDICAL ID

Wear medical identification at all times. Hypoglycemia can be mistaken for drunkenness. A medical ID tells strangers and emergency workers that you are probably having an insulin reaction. You can get necklaces, bracelets, sneaker tags, and watch charms. Emergency workers will probably look for neck chains and bracelets first. Also carry medical ID in your wallet.

LOWS AND ALCOHOL

When you're not eating (between meals and overnight), your liver releases glucose into your bloodstream. This gives you some protection from low blood glucose.

Your liver also has the job of clearing toxins from your blood. Alcohol is a toxin. When you drink alcohol, your liver gives priority to detoxifying your blood, and it doesn't release stored glucose. So alcohol increases the risk of hypoglycemia. Alcohol can contribute to a low even eight hours after your last drink. Physical activity when you're drinking, such as dancing, lowers blood glucose even more.

Current recommendations suggest that men keep their alcohol consumption to a maximum of two drinks a day and women keep their consumption to one drink a day. The standard advice is to drink only with meals. But this may not be enough to protect you from a low blood glucose episode. Alcohol's blocking effect on the liver lasts much longer than the glucose from your meal.

If you drink during the day, check your blood glucose level every two hours for eight hours. If it's low, eat a carbohydrate snack.

If you drink in the evening, keep track of the number of servings of alcohol you drink. Each of the following is one serving of alcohol:

- 12 oz of beer
- 4 oz of wine
- one shot of liquor

Before you go to bed, eat 10–15 grams of carbohydrate for each serving of alcohol you drank. If you normally eat a bedtime snack, eat your usual snack plus the extra carbohydrate. Eat this snack even if your blood glucose level is within or above your goal range (100–140 mg/dl for most people).

SUBJECT: I LIKE MY ALCOHOL

FROM: Sm

I like my alcohol. I have cut back to just a glass or two of wine at the most on weekends, but I know I am going to test the waters and have more than that soon. It seems to me my BS goes down when I drink. I am curious to know how alcohol affects diabetics. I am sure the answers will vary by person, but I would like to learn as much as possible before I find something out the hard way.

FROM: sh2

My endo told me a couple of glasses of wine, beer, or alcohol is okay, once in a while. I am on Lantus insulin and fast-acting Apidra before meals. Just make sure you eat something with your wine. And if on fast-acting, adjust accordingly, so you won't drop low.

FROM: A6

I too am a drinker, and sometimes definitely have more than two drinks. Education on your meds and how your liver works is VERY important if you are taking that chance. I always eat and take less insulin. I'd rather risk the high in the morning than the low while "not all there." I don't recommend it, but I know when I am out with friends it is just hard to stop at two. (That is an entirely different discussion!) Definitely talk to a diabetes educator and nutritionist.

FROM: Mo

My Dr. told me it was OK to have a drink or two if I followed the rules. Never drink on an empty stomach, test, eat carb-filled snacks to keep your sugar up, and have a glass of water between drinks.

FROM: tb

When I was newly dx even one or two beers on an empty stomach would drop my sugar low enough to cause shakes and mild vision problems. Now I eat before drinking and haven't had any problems.

FROM: lr

I take glipizide, and my numbers seem to be under control (14-day meter average: 84). I'm not a big drinker, but I do like to partake on some occasions. I asked my doctor if would be OK if I drank. He said that as long as I didn't drink on an empty stomach I should be OK. I ended up drinking, over a six-hour period, five low-carb beers and two shots of vodka. This was at a Christmas bowling party, and there was plenty of food to fill my stomach. To make a long story short, I woke up at 4:00 in the morning sweating, shaking, and my heart pounding. I took my BS, and it was at 40. I drank some orange juice and ate some crackers with peanut butter. This raised my BS into the low 60s. I don't think I will be drinking again!

9

Sick-Day Guidelines

The stress of an illness, wound, or infection makes your liver release glucose and makes your muscle and fat cells more resistant to insulin. So when you're sick, your blood glucose levels go up. Even an illness that doesn't keep you home sick in bed, such as a urinary tract infection, can make your blood glucose levels go up. If you are healing from a wound, that too can affect your blood glucose levels. Emotional stress can do the same thing.

SUBJECT: SCRAPES

FROM: gc

About three weeks ago, I fell while walking and scraped both my elbows bad enough that they were bleeding. I didn't think it was anything to worry about. I washed them, put on some Neosporin and bandages, and just went on about my business. The scrapes did not become infected, but they did take a little over a week to heal and there was some draining. During the healing period, my BG numbers went up quite a bit and I hadn't changed any of my eating habits. And of course seeing the numbers go up stressed me out. As soon as they healed, everything went back to where it had been before my fall.

It may seem that when you're so sick that you aren't eating or can't keep anything down, you shouldn't take your diabetes pills or insulin. But the opposite is true. You may need more insulin to control your blood glucose levels when you're sick.

BEFORE YOU GET SICK

Know what you need to do.

- Discuss sick-day management with your health care provider.
- Ask your spouse or other family member to go with you to this appointment. When all you want to do is lie in bed with the lights off, your spouse may be the one who will keep you from getting sicker by insisting that you eat, drink, check blood glucose levels and urine ketones, and call the doctor.

Ask your doctor about insulin.

- Your doctor may give you a sliding scale to use on sick days.

- If you're taking only basal insulin, you may need regular or rapid-acting insulin during an illness or infection. Your doctor may want to write a prescription for you now so you have it on hand for sick days.

Buy sick-day foods.

- You may want to keep these in a bag or box marked "Sick Day Foods." Put written instructions of what to do when you're sick and your doctor's phone and pager numbers inside.
- You can buy an over-the-counter electrolyte solution (balanced sugar-and-salt water) at your pharmacy or grocery store.
- Sports drinks, regular gelatin, regular soda, and bouillon cubes are also good.

SUBJECT: PNEUMONIA

FROM: gto

Hi everybody. Advice, please? I have developed pneumonia. My sugar numbers are usually in the normal range but are now very high. I was put on prednisone and puffers [inhaled steroids]. Could this be causing the big rise? Plus, I am getting very weak. Will be seeing my Doc on Thursday.

FROM: Gm2

In situations like this, my endo puts me on little bitty baby doses of before-meal insulin until I get over the steroids. Works great.

WHAT TO DO WHEN YOU ARE SICK

Know Your Diabetes Pills

- If you take metformin (Glucophage, Glucovance, Metaglip, Avandamet), call your doctor if you get sick, before taking your metformin. You may need to stop taking metformin until you're over your illness.
- Take your usual dose of other types of diabetes pills. If you can't keep the pills down, call your doctor.
- If your blood glucose level is below 70 mg/dl and your diabetes pills can cause hypoglycemia, first eat or drink something with carbohydrate, and then call your doctor.

Insulin

- You may need to take extra insulin when you're sick, even if you're not eating much.
- Follow the instructions of your health care provider.

Eat and Drink

Even if you're vomiting, have diarrhea, or your blood glucose level is high, take in at least 45–50 grams of carbohydrate every three to four hours (about 10–15 grams every hour).

15 Grams of Carbohydrate

1/2 cup regular soda
1 double Popsicle
1/2 cup regular gelatin
1 cup Gatorade
1 cup soup (not milk-based)
1 slice toast
6 soda crackers

Drink Plenty of Fluids

- To prevent dehydration, drink at least 8 oz (1 cup) of caffeine- and alcohol-free fluid every hour.
- You'll need some salt. Electrolyte solution, broth, and sports drinks have salt.
- If drinking makes you vomit, drink one to two tablespoons every 20 minutes or suck on a frozen pop.

Rest

- Give yourself permission to rest. The chores can wait.

Check Blood Glucose and Urine Ketones

- Check these levels at least every two to four hours, until the results are normal. (See p. 165 for more on ketones.)
- Set your alarm for the middle of the night and check then, too.

■ Call your doctor as needed. Don't wait until morning if your ketone or glucose levels are at dangerous levels.

Call Your Health Care Team

You should contact your health care provider when any of the following occur:

- Blood glucose is over 250 mg/dl for more than six hours.
- Blood glucose is over 350 mg/dl even once.
- Urine ketones are moderate or higher for more than six hours.
- You can't keep down any food or drink for more than four hours.
- You have a fever of over 101.5°F.
- Illness lasts more than 24 hours.
- You are dehydrated, have severe abdominal pain, or have other unexplained symptoms.

When you call, be ready to report your blood glucose level, ketone results, temperature, and symptoms. You can often reverse a moderately high blood glucose level at home. Your health care provider will give you instructions.

Get a Ride to the Hospital

■ A blood glucose level above 500 mg/dl is an emergency. Notify your doctor and have someone drive you to the hospital. Don't drive yourself—your thinking and reflexes may not be good.

WHEN YOU HAVE AN INFECTION

Your immune system is trying to fight the infection. White blood cells don't work well when glucose levels rise above 160 mg/dl, so keeping your blood glucose levels in the healthy ranges is a major goal when treating infections.

You may need to use more insulin than you normally take. As the infection comes under control, your blood glucose levels will start to drop, and you'll cut back on insulin. In the case of a foot ulcer that keeps you off your feet, you may need extra insulin until the infection is completely gone, the ulcer has healed, and you're back to your normal level of activity.

SUBJECT: FOOD POISONING

FROM: dec

I came down with a bad case of food poisoning (is there ever a good case?). By around 5:00 p.m., I was feeling queasy, so I checked my sugar. It was 190. About 8:00 p.m., the real heaves began. It didn't take much time before I realized I had food poisoning and not just a generic throw-up. By 10:15 p.m., BS 281. Left that alone because I was afraid that with such violent throwing up and no intake, it would drop like a rock on me. At 12:45 a.m., BS 354, so I stuck 15 units of Humalog (didn't take the 35 units of Lantus that I usually do or my 1,000 mg of metformin ER).

1:45 a.m.: BS 274.
2:50 a.m.: BS 345, so another 20 units of Humalog.
4:00 a.m.: BS 248.
5:45 a.m.: BS 235.
7:00 a.m.: BS 243.
10:30 a.m.: BS 232.

I had talked to my primary care doc around 10 a.m., and she agreed with my strategy to keep my BS higher because I could not keep anything down. Last throw-up was 7:00 a.m., and there had been some output on the other end. I had continued to drink as much water as I could through the night, knowing that I would return it, but hoping that I could retain just a little and not get dehydrated. Called out for Jesus quite a lot!

I could finally manage some vanilla yogurt about 11:00 a.m. and half a toasted English muffin by 1:00 p.m. Doctor advised me to eat a banana (woo-hoo!) to make sure that I hadn't lost any potassium.

This thing kicked my butt. I was out of work all week. I was so unexpectedly weak for a lot longer than I planned, and my brain absolutely turned to mush.

So, here's my cautionary tale. Even if you have food poisoning, you have to remember to be a "good" diabetic and remember to stick and test!

DIABETIC KETOACIDOSIS

Diabetic ketoacidosis (DKA) is usually associated with type 1 diabetes. But if you need insulin, you will need to think about many of the same things as do people with type 1 diabetes. You need to check for ketones when you are sick.

You know that insulin moves glucose into cells, and the cells use it for energy. When there isn't enough insulin, glucose can't move in, and cells are starved. So the body breaks down fat for energy. A byproduct of the breakdown of fat is ketones. If ketones form faster than the body can get rid of them, they build up in the blood. Ketones are acidic, and the blood starts to turn acidic.

Normally, people with type 2 diabetes make enough insulin to keep fats from breaking down. But when your body is under stress (an infection, a heart attack), your blood glucose levels will rise. If they're high enough for long enough, the insulin-producing cells of your pancreas shut down. They stop making insulin. Then ketones can build up.

The lack of insulin that leads to ketones also leads to high blood glucose levels, which leads to excess urination and dehydration. A buildup of ketones plus dehydration can lead to diabetic ketoacidosis (DKA). DKA can lead to coma and death.

Mild DKA can be treated at home with help from your diabetes educator or doctor. People with severe DKA need to be hospitalized. Treatment for DKA is insulin and fluids.

Symptoms of DKA	Signs that Others Might Notice
Nausea and vomiting	Warm, dry skin
Loss of appetite	Rapid breathing; sighing
Abdominal pain	Fruity odor on breath (like
Thirst	Juicy Fruit gum)
Weakness	
Visual disturbances	
Sleepiness	
Urinating a lot	

How to Check for Ketones

You can buy ketone strips at your pharmacy. You don't need a prescription. Don't wait until you're sick to get them. Keep them in your house and check the expiration date every six months.

When to Check for Ketones

- Several blood glucose tests in a day are 240 mg/dl or higher.
- You are sick or feel queasy. Ketones can make you feel sick to your stomach. Don't assume it's just something you ate or a 24-hour stomach flu.

Step-by-Step Procedure

Step 1. Dip a ketone test strip in a urine sample or pass it through the stream of urine.

Step 2. Time the test according to the directions on the package (10 seconds to two minutes, depending on the brand).

Step 3. There will be a color change if ketones are present. Compare the color on the strip to the package color chart and record the result. A result of "moderate" or "large" means you don't have enough insulin in your system. Call your doctor right away.

HIGH AND DRY: HHS

A combination of extremely high glucose levels (over 600 mg/dl) plus dehydration is an acute complication of type 2 diabetes called hyperosmolar hyperglycemic syndrome (HHS). It is also called hyperosmolar hyperglycemic nonketotic syndrome (HHNS). It is a life-threatening situation.

Anyone with type 2 diabetes can develop HHS, but it's not an everyday thing. Something starts the ball rolling: a urinary tract infection, pneumonia, an infection in the foot, a heart attack, or extensive burns. The stress of the illness or infection causes blood glucose levels to rise. Certain medications can also raise blood glucose levels. If blood glucose levels keep going up, you get glucose toxicity and dehydration. An illness that causes diarrhea or vomiting can cause you to lose even more fluid.

This may continue for days or weeks. You'll find yourself needing to urinate many times a day. You'll be very thirsty, but because of the loss of minerals with the urine, you may feel too weak to drink enough fluids. As your condition gets worse, you may stop feeling thirsty, possibly because the thirst center in your brain is affected. You will have a dry, parched mouth and throat and warm, dry skin (but no sweating).

Then you may start acting confused or sleepy. You may have a very high fever (for example, 105°F), loss of vision, or hallucinations. HHS is sometimes mistaken for a stroke because some people develop a weakness on one side of the body. Allowed to continue, the severe dehydration will lead to seizures, coma, and, eventually, death. As with DKA, treatment for HHS is insulin and IV fluids.

Signs and Symptoms of HHS
Dry, parched mouth
Warm, dry skin with no sweating
Extreme thirst (though this may gradually disappear)
Sleepiness or confusion
High blood glucose

Be Alert to HHS

A large number of medications have been reported to have caused hyperosmolar hyperglycemic syndrome on some occasions. One example is glucocorticoids ("steroids").

- Whenever you are prescribed a new medication, ask your pharmacist if it might affect your blood glucose levels.
- Check your blood glucose levels regularly for the first month that you're on a new medication, and tell your doctor about any unusual changes in your blood glucose levels.

About one-third of the cases of HHS occur in people living in nursing homes. If a loved one of yours is living in a nursing home and suddenly seems to be doing poorly, consider the possibility of HHS. If he or she is more confused than usual or appears to have had a stroke, insist that his or her blood glucose level be tested. People suffering from HHS can look deathly ill yet fully recover with treatment.

SUBJECT: STEROIDS

FROM: J14
I'm having an epidural injection of a steroid to help with the pain of sciatica today, and I know steroids increase BS and I will need to be especially careful.

My question is how long do the steroids from an injection affect blood sugar? Is it days, weeks, months?

FROM: R6

OMG, Kathy, I feel for ya. Been there for five years with the sciatic pain. I had six of the epidural injections. Oh yeah, steroids will jack up the blood sugar. I had an average of 275 for about a week before returning to what is normal for me. My brother had them as well. His lasted for about a week, too, although he ended up in the mid 300s. We both tried to counter the spikes by shooting more insulin and still had high numbers. The doctor told me that 5–10 days is the norm for the spikes.

FROM: D3

I had a steroid injection into my wrist last year, and it did not impact my BS all that much. Oral steroids are a whole different ballgame. They affect the entire body—not just one area—hence they can and do raise BS higher than would a localized injection.

FROM: J14

Thank you for your helpful info. I had the epidural yesterday and asked the doctor about how long my BS would be elevated. He said it should come back down in a couple days. It was 141 this morning, which is about 50 above my usual. I will just have to be very careful until it returns. He gave me 3/4 of the usual dose this time because of the BS problem.

10

Special Circumstances
Traveling, Pregnancy, and Religious Fasting

WHEN YOU TRAVEL

Before You Go

I f you'll be going overseas, make an appointment with your doctor or diabetes educator one to two months before you go. You'll want to discuss and develop plans to deal with the following issues.

Ask how to adjust your insulin plan and other diabetes medications.

- If you're on a split-mix plan, this may be a good time to switch to a flexible insulin plan.
- As you travel east, you lose time. If you keep taking insulin "on time" according to local clocks, you'll be bunching up your doses. You may need to take less insulin on the day you are crossing time zones. As you travel

---

west, you add hours to your day. You may need to take more insulin to cover this artificially long day. You may want to wait until you get to your final destination before you reset your watch.

Discuss sick-day management.
- If you are using only basal insulin, ask your doctor about getting one vial of regular or rapid-acting insulin, in case you get sick and need to control high glucose levels.

By Plane

When traveling by plane, pack your insulin and other diabetes supplies in your carry-on luggage. Checked luggage may get lost, and it's also subjected to extreme temperatures that are not good for your insulin or other supplies. Bring more diabetes supplies than you think you will need. Bring a second meter and batteries. Bring enough testing supplies to check your blood glucose every four to six hours, even if you don't check it that often at home.

For current information about taking your supplies through airport security, go to www.diabetes.org and search for "travel TSA." The TSA is the U.S. Transportation Security Administration, and it sets the rules for aviation security. Notify the screener that you have diabetes and are carrying your supplies with you. The TSA is not currently requiring prescription labels, but it recommends having the labels available in case there are any questions.

Bring your own food onto the plane. You should also bring glucose tabs or other treatments for low blood glucose. If you also buy food on board, don't take your mealtime insulin until the food is in front of you. The food cart could be one row away from you when the plane hits turbulence, and you may never get your meal.

Drink plenty of fluids, but avoid alcohol. Alcohol can lead to unexpected lows (p. 153). You'll have enough affecting your blood glucose levels without adding alcohol to the mix.

If you draw up insulin when you're in the air, you may not have to inject air first because of pressure differences (see Preparing the Syringe, p. 208).

Prescriptions

When traveling, it's best to bring all the insulin you will need. Just in case, also bring your prescriptions for insulin and syringes or bring the prescription label. If you run out, a local pharmacist can contact your doctor or original pharmacy and get you what you need.

Activity

Strolling through quaint towns, going on walking tours of historic sites, pacing in the airport when the flight is delayed . . . people are usually much more active than usual when they're traveling. Physical activity increases your insulin sensitivity. You may experience low blood glucose. Check your blood glucose levels every four to six hours while you're traveling. Always carry snacks and glucose tabs or hard candy.

Wear medical ID. Tell your traveling companions and tour director that you have diabetes and explain the symptoms and treatment of low blood glucose.

Check your feet every day when you're traveling. (This is for anyone who has diabetes, whether on insulin or not.) At the slightest problem, even just a red spot that doesn't fade away, stay off your feet the next day. Because you have diabetes, even a small blister can turn into a much bigger problem if you keep walking on it.

PREGNANCY

Your baby's organs form during the first six to eight weeks after conception. If your blood glucose levels are close to the normal, nondiabetic range during this time, your baby's risk of birth defects is almost as low as that for the infant of a mother who doesn't have diabetes. Blood glucose levels in the normal range throughout your pregnancy will help keep your baby from growing too large (a condition called macrosomia).

See your doctor six months before you start trying to get pregnant. You'll likely need a change in your insulin plan to get the near-normal glucose levels you want for conception, and you'll want your new diabetes plan to be second nature by the time you conceive. Your doctor may have you stop taking all of your diabetes pills and go on a basal-bolus insulin plan.

SUBJECT: PLANNING TO GET PREGNANT

FROM: wh2

My husband and I would like to have another child. I know that once I get pregnant I will have to switch from meds to insulin. Here are my questions:

1) Will my baby be in any kind of risk with me having diabetes?
2) If I were to get pregnant while taking my meds (metformin, glipizide, Actos), can any of these meds (or all of them) affect my baby?
3) Is it possible to not be on any kind of meds—including insulin—while pregnant? Hopefully, someone who's had this experience can give me a little insight.

FROM: cd10

I have type 2 and am on my third pregnancy since dx. I was actually diagnosed during my second pregnancy. Unfortunately, since I did not know I had diabetes when I first became pregnant and my A1C was

9.5, I had a miscarriage. The loss of my pregnancy put me in a deep depression for months. Fortunately, I got my sugars under decent control with only diet control. I lost about 40 pounds and found out a year after I lost my second child that I was pregnant again. My A1C at that time was 6.2 (anything under 7% gives you a better chance for a healthy pregnancy and less chance for birth defects), and I was immediately put on insulin. Oral meds are not allowed during pregnancy because they can damage the fetus. It has something to do with the way the meds are filtered through the placenta. I don't think it is possible to go without insulin because of the effects pregnancy has on your BS. In fact, the farther along you get in your pregnancy, the more insulin you have to take. I have to give myself shots four times per day.

Anyway, the biggest risks to the baby apart from birth defects and miscarriage because of poor BS control prior to and at the beginning of pregnancy are low blood sugars, underdeveloped lungs, and shoulder dystocia.

I, unfortunately, decided that since I was on insulin, I didn't have to control my diet as much as before. My son weighed nine pounds, four ounces at birth. Because of his size, his shoulder became caught on my pelvic bone during birth (shoulder dystocia). I hope this information helped a little, and good luck to you!

FROM: TK

My husband and I are talking about having another baby in the near future and this is the advice I was given by my doctor. He told me that I should stop the metformin and go on insulin before becoming pregnant. He also wants me to have at least two A1Cs lower than 6% before attempting. I am on birth control for now. As soon as my A1Cs are down and we decide to go ahead and I stop the birth control, I am supposed to immediately switch to insulin. I had gestational diabetes with our son, and all I can tell you is to be very strict about your BG control. I wasn't so good about mine the first time, and my son ended up being born six weeks premature (weighing 5 1/2 pounds!!!). I would have had a 10-pound baby if he had been full term. He had a three-week stay in the NICU but has no health problems now. Diabetes educators are wonderful and offered me a lot of great advice when I was pregnant.

Oh, and another thing, you will probably have to have regular fetal stress tests and sonograms in the end stages of your pregnancy. I had to go twice a week while they attached me to a fetal heart monitor and had me mark when he moved. They also checked my amniotic fluid levels regularly through ultrasound because people with diabetes can have low fluid levels. You will have check-ups more often than someone who isn't diabetic and will probably see a high-risk obstetrician. I actually enjoyed the time off my feet. Good luck.

FROM: hp1
I used to work in high-risk pregnancies, labor, and delivery, so I want to emphasize some things. You

must have excellent control of your blood sugars for several months before trying for a baby, hence the statement about having at least two good A1C tests (representing six months). The damage to the baby mostly occurs VERY early in pregnancy, well before you are aware that you are pregnant. I STRONGLY urge you and anyone else who is thinking about having a baby to see a high-risk pregnancy specialist (perinatologist) and a diabetes doctor (endocrinologist) at least a year before you try to conceive. Having expert advice, as close to perfect blood sugar control as you can get, and taking a prenatal vitamin with folic acid will greatly increase your chances of having a healthy baby. I have been out of the field for several years now and don't know the up-to-the-minute info about meds and pregnancy, but I do know that insulin is the gold standard of maintaining BS control while pregnant. I think that there's research showing some oral meds may be safe, but I don't know the details. Good luck!

FROM: rp

Like one of the other posters, I've also had a miscarriage caused by uncontrolled BS levels, right after dx, at nine weeks. So getting your levels under control before conception is crucial. From conception to about 12 weeks is the most critical period of development. Keeping your levels in control during this time will give you an excellent chance for a healthy baby. As far as insulin goes, yes, you will probably have to switch to it. Consider using the pump instead of injections. If mine had continued, I would've gone to it for convenience and better control. Best of luck to you!

RELIGIOUS FASTING: RAMADAN

Worldwide, many religions use fasting as a means of worship. Millions of people with diabetes throughout the world fast during Ramadan. The Koran exempts the sick from the duty of fasting, especially if it might lead to harm, and people with diabetes fall into this group. Still, many people with diabetes insist on fasting. This creates a medical challenge for themselves and their health care providers.

There have been few studies on the effects of fasting in people with diabetes. The American Diabetes Association convened a group of 15 endocrinologists and diabetologists from a number of Muslim and non-Muslim countries to look at the issue. Here is a summary of the risks of fasting for people with type 2 diabetes and the group's recommendations.

Major Risks of Fasting

Hypoglycemia (Low Blood Glucose)

The Epidemiology of Diabetes and Ramadan (EPIDIAR) study included 12,243 people with diabetes from 13 Islamic countries. It showed that fasting during Ramadan increased the risk of severe low blood glucose requiring hospitalization in people with type 2 diabetes.

Hyperglycemia (High Blood Glucose)
The EPIDIAR study showed a fivefold increase in severe high blood glucose requiring hospitalization in people with type 2 diabetes. Some people may have reduced the dosage of their diabetes medications too much in an effort to avoid hypoglycemia.

Dehydration and Blood Clots
Limiting fluids for a long time can lead to dehydration. This may become severe in hot and humid climates. People who do hard physical labor also lose fluid through sweat. If blood glucose levels are too high, the body will put out more urine. People with diabetes already have blood that is prone to clotting, which can lead to heart attack and stroke. Dehydration raises the risk of clots. However, two studies did not show an increase in hospitalizations due to heart problems or stroke during Ramadan.

Your Risk

Because you use insulin, you don't fall into the "low risk" or "moderate risk" groups. Your risk of developing problems during a fast may put you in the "high risk" or "very high risk" groups. People at high risk include those with high blood glucose (A1C over 7.5%), those with other medical problems, and those who live alone. Discuss your risks with your health care provider. The advice will probably be not to fast.

Fasting during pregnancy would be expected to carry a high risk of health problems and even death for the fetus and mother. Pregnant Muslim women are exempt from fasting during Ramadan, but some insist on fasting. They need intensive diabetes care. Ideally, they should be managed in high-risk clinics staffed by obstetricians, diabetologists, nutritionists, and diabetes nurse educators.

Before Ramadan

If you are determined to fast, see your doctor one to two months before Ramadan. Ask about your risks based on your medical history. Your doctor may order blood work. If you both decide that you may be able to fast without too much risk, discuss what your diabetes care plan will be.

Insulins that peak during the fast may cause problems. A study on fasting was done using insulin glargine, which has little to no peak. In 15 people with well-controlled type 1 diabetes who fasted for 18 hours (not for Ramadan), the average blood glucose dropped from 125 to 93 mg/dl during the fast. Two episodes of mild hypoglycemia occurred. The duration of the fast in Ramadan is typically less than 18 hours, so this study suggests that one option would be to use a peakless basal insulin and premeal rapid-acting insulin.

You should also see your diabetes educator. You and your family should review:

- signs and symptoms of high and low blood glucose
- treatment of highs and lows
- blood glucose monitoring
- meal planning
- effects of physical activity

During Ramadan

- Wear a medical alert ID, such as a bracelet.
- Check your blood glucose levels several times every day.
- Drink plenty of fluids during the hours when you don't fast.
- Eat the predawn meal as late as possible, before the start of the daily fast.
- Exercise normally.
  - Avoid excessive physical activity. This could lead to low blood glucose, particularly during the few hours before the sunset meal.
  - If Tarawih prayer (multiple prayers after the sunset meal) is done, count it as part of your daily exercise program.

- Break the fast if you need to.
  - You must end your fast right away if your blood glucose goes below 60 mg/dl. If you wait or delay treatment, your blood glucose could drop even lower.
  - Break the fast if your blood glucose drops to less than 70 mg/dl in the first few hours after the start of the fast, especially if you took insulin, a sulfonylurea, or a meglitinide (Starlix or Prandin) at predawn.
  - Break the fast if your blood glucose goes above 300 mg/dl.
  - Do not fast if you're sick.

After Ramadan

Your overall doses of medications, especially insulin, will need to be adjusted if you gain or lose weight during Ramadan.

11

How To
From Buying to Injecting

SUBJECT: ANNOYED

FROM: KQ

When I went on Lantus, my doctor gave me the Rx and made an appointment for me to return and have the nurse show me how to use it. She gave me about a two-minute lesson. She even used a regular syringe for the demonstration but told me my syringe would be smaller and different. When I asked about syringes, she gave me an Rx for that.

When I got to the pharmacy, they asked ME what kind of syringes I used. The Rx just said "insulin syringes." I said, "No clue." Thankfully, together we figured it out. I then went to the home of a friend who has diabetes, and SHE actually showed me how to do it.

LEARNING HOW TO USE INSULIN

Many people with type 2 diabetes see primary care providers, not diabetes specialists. Primary care staff may not have a lot of experience teaching people how to use insulin. Even if you do see an endocrinologist, the appointment may not last long enough for you to ask all your questions and get comfortable with injecting.

See a Certified Diabetes Educator

The best thing you can do for yourself is to make an appointment with a certified diabetes educator. Medicare covers these sessions (see p. 188), and so do many private insurance plans. Ask your doctor for a referral. To find an educator near you, go to the American Association of Diabetes Educators at www.aadenet.org and click on "Find an Educator."

Prep Before You Go

You'll get more from your appointment with your CDE if you go in with some preparation. Four companies (Eli Lilly, Novo Nordisk, Sanofi-Aventis, and Pfizer) distribute insulins in the U.S. Their websites have instructions on how to use their insulins and their insulin pens. Some have videos with narration. A syringe manufacturer (BD) also has video animation on how to draw up insulin and how to inject. These videos are far better than anything we can do here in print. If you don't have a computer at home, consider using one at your local library or senior center.

Websites with Instructions on Using Insulin

Eli Lilly	www.lillydiabetes.com
	www.humalog.com
Novo Nordisk	www.novonordisk-us.com
	www.novolog.com
	www.levemir-us.com
Sanofi-Aventis	www.sanofi-aventis.com/us
	www.lantus.com
	www.apidra.com
Pfizer (inhaled insulin)	www.exubera.com
BD Diabetes Learning Center	www.bddiabetes.com/us

For information on hundreds of diabetes products, including syringes, injection aids, insulin pens, and insulin pumps, see the American Diabetes Association's annual Resource Guide. You can find it in the January issue of *Diabetes Forecast* or go to www.diabetes.org and search "Resource Guide."

MEDICARE COVERAGE FOR DIABETES SELF-MANAGEMENT TRAINING

By Peggy Bourgeois, APRN, MN, CNS, CDE

Your doctor says you need to start on insulin. He doesn't have time in a regular appointment to teach you everything you need to get started, so he tells you to see a diabetes educator. And you think, "Yikes, what will that cost?"

If you're on Medicare, it should cost you only your co-pay. On February 1, 2001, Centers for Medicare and Medicaid Services (CMS) began covering outpatient diabetes self-management training (DSMT). Many private plans have followed suit.

CMS requires that you go to a DSMT program that meets certain quality standards that have been approved by a national accreditation organization. Currently, CMS recognizes the American Diabetes Association (ADA) and the Indian Health Service (IHS) as approved national accreditation organizations. Diabetes programs that have not received certification or accreditation by either of these organizations will not receive payment by CMS. To find an ADA-certified program near you, call 1-800-DIABETES (1-800-342-2383).

Medicare will cover DSMT services only if the health care professional who is managing your diabetes and who is a Medicare provider refers you for the services. Over the course of your lifetime, you are eligible for:

- one 10-hour initial training within a 12-month period
- two hours of DSMT every 12 months thereafter

Your health care provider orders the initial training, which includes a one-hour, one-on-one visit and up to nine hours of group training. If you have a limitation that would make group training difficult for you, such as a vision, hearing, physical, language, or cognitive impairment, your provider can order individual training for you in place of the group training.

ADDITIONAL TRAINING

You may be able to get additional DSMT if there is a significant change in your treatment plan, such as "change in medication to insulin due to excessive hyperglycemia." CMS does not state how many additional hours will be approved.

Even with a referral, don't be surprised if CMS denies these additional hours of DSMT when the bill is first submitted. You should file an appeal with CMS. Often patients throw their hands up in disgust, thinking, "What's the use? They're going to deny it anyway." Writing a letter of appeal is not a waste of time. CMS denies many claims at first and then approves the charges upon receiving letters of appeal. The DSMT program manager will be willing to assist you in your appeal, which should include:

- a letter from your health care provider stating the reasons why additional training was needed
- a copy of the referral form
- a letter of appeal from the diabetes educator and/or you
- copies of blood glucose levels and A1C values, weight loss/gain, blood pressure changes, abnormal cholesterol, or triglycerides
- number of past hospitalizations or emergency room visits for high or low blood glucose levels

LIMITS ON COVERAGE

Remember, there is a limit to the number of hours of DSMT that you can get under Medicare. It begins within any month of the year following the referral, for the upcoming 12-month period. Don't procrastinate. You must attend the program during the 12 months following the referral. Medicare will not give you another 12 months to make up the 10-hour program.

If your health care provider refers you for an initial 10-hour DSMT program but you have already attended a 10-hour program as a Medicare beneficiary, you will be denied coverage for another 10-hour program. The benefit for two additional hours must occur in the following calendar year (January to December) following the last hour of DSMT you attended. Otherwise, the two hours of additional training will be denied. Medicare scans the referral into their computer system to track the number of hours of DSMT you have received.

However, if you attended a DSMT program before becoming a Medicare beneficiary, you may attend another 10-hour program after becoming a Medicare beneficiary. Also, if you were a Medicare beneficiary and attended a DSMT program before February 2001, you may receive one full 10-hour DSMT program after February 2001 because CMS did not have provisions for DSMT prior to February 2001.

What if you don't know how many hours of DSMT you are eligible for because you attended a "few" hours of a program several months or years ago? Call Medicare at 1-800-633-4227, tell them you need to know how many hours of Diabetes Self-Management Training you are eligible for or how many hours are on your record or account. Give your name, social security number, date of birth, and G0108 and/or G0109 codes that would have been used in billing your account. CMS will give you the exact number of hours you have been billed for. Your doctor may refer you to a program that will ask you for this information. Why? If you are billed for more than the 10-hour initial DSMT or two-hour annual, the program will not be paid for their services and neither can they bill you for services rendered. If you are not eligible for DSMT services, you will be asked to read and sign an Advanced Beneficiary Notice (ABN), which informs you that you will be responsible for the bill, the reason for denial such as, "used initial 10-hr DSMT time," and the exact amount you will be charged. You may choose to sign or not to sign the ABN.

DSMT is the best benefit CMS offers for people with diabetes, yet many people don't use it. Take advantage of the opportunity to learn everything you can about this disease from health care professionals who teach it. Be a partner with your diabetes care team and work with them to keep yourself healthy now and in the years to come.

Peggy Bourgeois, APRN, MN, CNS, CDE, is president of PBB Associates, LLC, Consultant Clinical Diabetes Education and Research. She was the director of the Diabetes Center of the Baton Rouge General Medical Center for 23 years. This is adapted from an article that appeared in Diabetes Spectrum *(18:62–64, 2005).*

GADGETS TO MAKE YOUR LIFE EASIER

Ask your diabetes educator or pharmacist to show you the injection aids described in this section.

Automatic injectors are good if you don't want to see a needle or if you have arthritis or problems holding a syringe steady. You hold the automatic injector to your skin, push a button, and the spring-loaded device inserts a needle into your skin. Some automatically release the insulin when the needle enters the skin. With others, you have to press the plunger on the syringe.

FROM: E7
I use this to inject myself about six times per day. If it is a fear of pushing the needle into yourself, this is the answer.

Dose gauges help you measure insulin accurately, even mixed doses. Some sound a click with every 1–2 units of insulin; others have Braille or raised numbers.

Needle guides, vial stabilizers, and **syringe guides** help you insert the needle into the insulin vial or draw out a set dose.

Syringe magnifiers enlarge the measure marks on an insulin syringe barrel.

Insulin Pens

Insulin pens are popular because they deliver accurate doses and are convenient. With an insulin pen, you don't have to fill a syringe. You either load a 3-ml (300-unit) cartridge of insulin into a reusable pen or you buy prefilled, disposable pens. You attach a pen needle, dial in your dose, and inject. Then you take the needle off and store the pen until its next use.

Pen needles of different lengths and gauge (a measure of how thin the needle is) are available. See ADA's Resource Guide for descriptions, and ask your diabetes educator for advice on which type would be best for you. It's important to take the needle off (and dispose of it) after each use. If you left the needle on, insulin could leak out or air could leak into the insulin cartridge, which could lead to inaccurate doses or contamination.

Most insulins are available in prefilled pens or in cartridges for pen use. (The exceptions are Humulin

R, Humulin 50/50, and U-500 Humulin R.) If your pen contains NPH or a premix, remember to mix the insulin thoroughly by tilting and rolling the pen each time before you use it.

SUBJECT: MORE PRAISE FOR PENS

FROM: D

I use needle and vial for the Lantus. I also have NovoLog for spikes over 200 (never needed that except once early on and again after the steroids, but love having it handy), and for NovoLog I do use the pen. It is VERY easy, just dial up the units instead of messing with and "eyeballing" the syringe. It is so easy to use the pen. My 8-year-old niece gave me a shot with it!

FROM: pj

When injecting, remember to keep the needle in for 10 seconds after injection to make sure it is all dispersed. You can tell it has when you take it out and it does not continue to bead up at the tip. I usually count to 15 just to be sure I got it all.

FROM: ja8

So now I am insulin dependent. I'm OK with it as long as it works. I don't have a problem giving myself a shot. But what is getting on my nerves is the time it takes. I have to do the whole testing shot production all the time. I went out and got a bigger purse, but now it weighs like 1,000 pounds. I couldn't imagine carrying that thing around the mall. So I was just wondering how you all haul your testing and insulin supplies with you all the time.

FROM: tia

I use Lantus and NovoLog, too. If you haven't tried them—try the pens. I find the NovoLog pen to be much more convenient than vials and syringes—mostly when I'm out and about. I also waste less insulin this way, too. Each cartridge is good for 28 days—same as a vial. This all depends on the amount you take as well as on your insurance co-pay, but it may be cheaper because of less waste. One box of Lantus cartridges lasts me over three months—for the same co-pay as one vial!

FROM: VV

I must agree. The pen sure does make life easier. I have been using Lantus from a vial (because they ran out of pens at my Dr's office). My evening injection is quite the little production. I get out my little box of syringes, my little box of alcohol wipes, my vial of Lantus, measure up, make sure I have just the right amount of insulin, tap out the bubbles, etc., etc.

Today they put me on Humalog (in addition to the Lantus) and that is in a pen. I couldn't believe how easy it was! By the way, also got my OptiClik pen for the Lantus today. Why, it was like a medical supply Christmas. I walked out of there with a box of this, a box of that, and a bag of this and that.

The Humalog and Lantus pens both take the same needle tips and fit nicely into the one carrying case that came with the Humalog. And the case is not really any bigger than my glucose meter.

The only thing that I still need is a personal assistant to tell me how much to take. I am feeling a little overwhelmed by the "if it is this number to that number take this many units 15 minutes BEFORE you eat" and "if it is this number to that number take this many units 15 minutes AFTER you eat" and "if it is this number to that number take this many units AS you begin to eat." I made up a little cheat sheet to carry in my insulin case.

I really think I am ready for managed care. You know, where someone takes care of my everyday needs. Bring me just the right amount of medicine just when I need it. Bring me my diabetes-friendly meals and snacks in just the right-sized servings for me at just the right time. Take me to my exercise every day. I could be such a good diabetes patient that way.

BUYING INSULIN

Older insulins don't require a prescription, but the newer insulins do. But you really need a prescription no matter what type of insulin you use, for insurance coverage and to avoid mistakes (Humulin vs. Humalog, Novolin 70/30 vs. NovoLog 70/30).

You can buy insulin at an independent pharmacy, a chain pharmacy, or through mail order. Some people like the personal touch and get to know their pharmacists. A pharmacist can become another member of your diabetes care team. Indeed, some are certified diabetes educators. You can ask questions, find out about new products, and see the latest gadgets.

Some people prefer to use a chain pharmacy so that when they travel, they can get supplies easily through computer transfer of the prescription.

Yet other people prefer to use mail order pharmacies or are required to by their insurance plan. Insulin spoils if it gets colder than 36°F or hotter than 86°F, and refrigeration (36–46°F) is always preferred. Consider the temperatures your insulin will be subjected to in transit and while sitting in your mailbox or on your front porch. Ask the distributor how the insulin is protected. Check all the insulin vials when you open the box and make sure the insulin looks normal.

You may get a discount for buying certain quantities at your pharmacy or by mail order. If you are buying in bulk, make sure to check the expiration date. Make sure you'll use the insulin before it expires.

If you're buying at a pharmacy, bring along an empty vial to make sure you get exactly the same thing each time.

SUBJECT: DESERT LIVING

FROM: Rz

I get my meds through the mail. It's cheaper for me that way. Just started this, by the way. WELL, yesterday my insulin (three vials) came in an envelope, with no ice pack. I live in the desert. Can you imagine how hot they were? I can't believe people in the pharmacy could be so dumb. It must be assistants that pack it; however, you'd think they would be better informed. Tried to call them right away. Of course, they are closed on the weekends. Speak of frustration!!!

FROM: hp1
I would be SERIOUSLY aggravated and demanding a cold-packed replacement sent by overnight FedEx.

HOW TO STORE INSULIN

Unopened, refrigerated insulin that has not been mishandled in transit is good until its expiration date. Keep insulin in the back of your refrigerator (but not under the vent that leads from the freezer) and in the box so it's protected from light. If you store insulin in a cooler on a trip, make sure it doesn't touch ice or freeze.

Once a vial or pen has been used once, the clock starts. A vial of insulin is good for 28–42 days, depending on the type of insulin and the brand. In-use cartridges and prefilled pens are good for 10–42 days, depending on the type and brand. Check the instructions on your insulin. Storage and in-use times can be different even within insulin "families." For example, one brand of rapid-acting insulin in a pen is good for 28 days, but that same brand of rapid-acting insulin in a premix in a pen is good for only 10 days. Recheck the instructions every once in a while. Recommendations from the manufacturers sometimes change as they do more testing.

Take a Look at Your Insulin

When you take out a new vial, cartridge, or pen, inspect it to make sure that it looks okay.

- Glargine, detemir, regular, and the rapid-acting insulins are clear. Check for particles or discoloration. Any cloudiness may mean that the insulin is contaminated and you shouldn't use it.
- NPH and premixed insulins are suspensions. After they are gently remixed (by rolling and turning over) they should look uniformly cloudy. Don't use insulin that has "frosting" inside or large clumps floating in it. These changes mean crystals are forming. This can be caused by shaking or by letting the insulin get too hot or too cold.

Get the Most from Your Insulin

- A vial may last you a long time. Write the date you start on the vial.
- Throw the insulin away when you get to the end of the use-by time. There may be a noticeable drop in effectiveness if you use the insulin after this time.
- Some manufacturers recommend you keep an in-use vial refrigerated; others say room temperature is fine for their products.
- Keep in-use pens at room temperature.
- Don't let insulin sit in direct sun or in your car on a hot day.

Insulin can go bad if it sits in the sun, freezes, gets too warm, is shaken too much, or is too old. There may not be a visible change in the insulin. If your blood glucose levels are high for no apparent reason, consider starting a new vial of insulin.

SUBJECT: AFTER 28 DAYS . . .

FROM: cb

I will be starting Lantus tomorrow (it's in the fridge as we speak). I've heard that it's good for 28 days after opening, but I have enough for something like 200 injections—do you just throw it out after 28 days?

FROM: tmp

Yes, you do have to throw it out after approximately 28 days. You will find that it loses its effectiveness approximately 28 days after you open it. Sometimes I forget to mark the date of opening, and about a month later I'll notice that my morning BG numbers are suddenly higher. I'll open a new vial that night to use—voilà—my numbers are back down the next morning.

FROM: D

Hey girl, welcome to the Lantus Club. I do toss any leftover insulin after 28 days. If you are using a tiny amount, it might be more cost-effective for you to get the pen vials. There are only 3 ml in each of those. You get five in a box (15 ml) for the same co-pay, and each one can be used for 28 days. Don't be surprised when your dose goes up for a while until you get it where it needs to be, though.

SUBJECT: REFRIGERATE?

FROM: DJ

I have type 2 and take Lantus insulin (70 units) every night before going to bed. Some nights when giving myself the shot, it stings while injecting the insulin. Is this normal? Why does it happen only once in a while? I do rotate locations, though I do use my abdomen as my primary location. Other locations hurt more and/or difficult to reach. Any suggestions?

FROM: tmp

Is the Lantus cold or room temperature? Some people find it more painful if it is cold. Also, it is possible that you are hitting a small vein or something. Sometimes mine stings, sometimes it doesn't. These are the suggestions I've gotten in the past, but for me, it seems like it's just luck of the draw (ha ha).

FROM: DJ

The Lantus is right from the refrigerator so it is cold, but not too cold. It's just weird how sometimes it stings, while most of the time it does not. I thought maybe I was doing something wrong while injecting, etc. Where do you give yourself the shots?

FROM: tmp

My abdomen, which seems to have the best subcutaneous fat—at least it is quite plentiful! I've also used my thighs, when I get sick of too many bruises on my tummy (I bruise easily). Actually, less sting or discomfort in my thigh, but I've heard that the abdomen is still the best place. You might try not keeping it in the fridge. It should be stored in the fridge before the vial is opened, but once it is opened it doesn't need refrigeration—it stays good for 28 days. I find it more comfortable at room temperature.

FROM: DJ

I am looking at my Lantus insulin box, and it says to "keep refrigerated."

FROM: tmp

While it does say to keep refrigerated, you'll notice that it also says it can be kept unrefrigerated for up to 28 days after opening. That's why I don't even bother to refrigerate once it is opened anymore, and its effectiveness is just fine.

FROM: D

I keep mine refrigerated, fill the syringe, and just let THAT warm a bit before using it.

FROM: tia

The OptiClik pen device can NOT be stored in the fridge (something about the electronic parts), so I leave my opened cartridge at room temperature, and it's fine.

FROM: VY

I too have found some injections sting but most don't. I figured it was just what I was hitting when I injected. My first vial was kept at room temperature after opening per my doctor's instructions. He also told me to use my syringes more than once (unlike the package instructions). I keep my second vial in the fridge. I like keeping it in the fridge.

FROM: Dvd

I read through the thread and have not seen this suggestion. Make sure the alcohol has dried after you prep the skin. I find that I get in a hurry sometimes, and this will sting for about 10 seconds or so.

I have also hit a vein, and it causes a small pain that is almost instantly over. I have no idea how to avoid that, it just seems to happen sometimes.

SYRINGES

You'll buy syringes with needles already attached. Syringes come in a variety of sizes (the volume that they hold). Your syringe needs to be large enough to hold your entire dose but small enough that reading the marking scale is easy. Look at several brands of syringe. One might be easier for you to handle or to see the markings.

Depending on how much the syringe holds, each line means a different amount of insulin.

If Your Syringe Holds This Much . . .	Its Capacity Is . . .	Each Line Means . . .
1 cc	100 units	2 units
1/2 cc	50 units	1 unit
3/10 cc	30 units	1 or 1/2 unit (check the instructions)

You have different options for both needle length (5/16″, 3/8″, or 1/2″) and needle diameter (gauge, or G). Your options are 28G, 29G, 30G, 31G; the higher the gauge, the thinner the needle (31G is thinner than 30G). Ask your diabetes educator what size needle is best for your body type.

When traveling, take enough supplies plus a doctor's prescription for syringes and your prescription label. In some states, you may not be able to get your syringes without a prescription. If you run out, a local pharmacist can contact your doctor or pharmacy. If you run into problems, try a hospital emergency room.

SUBJECT: BUMPS AND BRUISES FROM INJECTIONS

FROM: 5c

I just started taking Lantus. Not sure I am doing it correctly. I am getting bumps and bruises at injection sites. Should this be happening?

FROM: mes

I give my grandfather injections in his arms in the back fatty part. I found if I pinch the skin together and inject the Lantus, I am less likely to get the bump and bruise. I did find when first giving the injection that I was getting the bumps and bruises. I count out how many units are going in, so I know it is going in slowly. Good luck. Hope this helps.

FROM: D

The bruises generally mean you hit a capillary (small blood vessel) and isn't a big deal medically, it just looks bad. Same thing if you get a drop of blood leaking out when you withdraw the needle. Not sure about the bumps . . . maybe it isn't absorbing very fast?

Do you use the regular or short needles? I have fewer bruises since I switched to short.

Also, I take 44 units. I've learned these few things.

1. Fill the syringe and let it warm in your hand for a minute or two before injecting. Cuts down on the "afterburn."
2. Inject no more than 15 units, then count slowly to at least 10 before injecting another 15 units. When you empty the syringe, count to at least 20 before withdrawing.
3. If anything seeps out, put your finger there and hold it for 20 count, don't press hard, just block the hole.

FROM: T
I have been using Lantus for over a year now and have not had that kind of problem. I use a 30-gauge needle, 1/2″, and inject it into my belly (60 units at bedtime). I think you should let your health care provider know that you are having this kind of reaction and let them advise you as to what to do.

FROM: hp1
Don't rub the site of the injection afterwards. Put firm, steady pressure on the site for 30–60 seconds. That will allow the blood to start to clot and reduce risk of bruises. Good luck!

INSULIN INJECTIONS: STEP BY STEP

Preparing the Syringe

Supplies
- A sterile syringe.
- Insulin vial. Check that the insulin looks normal.
- Alcohol swab.

Instructions
1. Wash your hands.
2. With NPH or a premixed insulin, you have to remix it before you use it. Roll the insulin vial between your hands 10 times and turn it over 10 times. Don't shake it because that makes bubbles in the insulin and then you can't measure the correct dose of insulin.

3. Wipe the vial stopper with an alcohol pad. (The first time you use a vial, remove the flat cap, but leave the metal ring and stopper. Write the current date on the outside of the vial to record when it was first opened.)

4. Hold the syringe with the needle pointing up. Fill it with air equal to the dose of insulin.

5. Remove the cover from the needle. Put the insulin vial on a table, holding it firmly, and push the needle into the rubber cover of the insulin vial. Inject the air into the vial. This makes it easier to extract the insulin.

6. Leave the needle in the vial with the plunger pushed in and turn over the vial. The needle should be covered with insulin.

7. Draw the correct dose of insulin into the syringe.

8. Check whether there are air bubbles inside the syringe. If you see bubbles (and if you haven't mixed insulins in this syringe), with the needle in the vial, hold the vial straight up and tap until the bubbles float. Push them out with the plunger and draw in the correct dose.

9. Take the needle out of the vial. Check again to see you have the correct dose of insulin.

10. If you have to put the syringe down before giving yourself the injection, make sure the needle doesn't touch anything, and put the cap on.

How to Mix NPH with Rapid-Acting or Regular Insulin

Supplies
- A new, sterile syringe of the correct size for the total combined units of insulin.
- Vial of each type of insulin you need.

Instructions
1. Make sure you know how much of each insulin you need and the total combined units you need. Add: the units of rapid or regular insulin plus the units of NPH.
2. Wash your hands.
3. Roll the vial of NPH between your hands 10 times and turn it over 10 times. Don't shake it.
4. Draw air into the syringe equal to the dose of NPH.
5. Hold the vial on the table and inject air into the vial. Remove the needle without removing any insulin.
6. Draw air into the syringe equal to the dose of regular or rapid insulin and inject air into the vial of regular or rapid insulin.
7. With the needle still inside the vial of regular or rapid insulin, turn the vial upside down to cover the whole needle with insulin.
8. Draw in the correct dose of insulin. Check for bubbles. Remove the needle.

9. With the vial of NPH on the table, insert the syringe. (You should already have injected air into the insulin vial.)

10. Turn the vial upside down and slowly draw in the exact dose of NPH. Remember to pull back the plunger to **the total combined number of units**.

11. Make sure again that you have the correct dose of insulin. If you have taken out too much insulin, throw the syringe away and start over. Do not return any insulin you have left over into this vial, because it's now a mixture.

How to Give Yourself an Injection

Sites You Can Use
- Abdomen. This is the best place. With some insulins, absorption is different at the different sites. The abdomen gives the most consistent absorption. Inject anywhere except within an inch of your navel.
- Arm. In the back part of your upper arm, where there is the most fat.
- Thighs, but not the insides.
- Buttocks.

SUBJECT: WHERE DO YOU INJECT?

FROM: E7
I usually inject into my stomach because this really hurts the least.

FROM: jz

I find my stomach area easiest.

FROM: cb

I got very sick and was in and out of the hospital because of my fear of needles. I was not going to stick myself in the stomach. No way. So I started by using the outer portion of my thigh, and I switch back and forth each day. I could deal with a thigh because it's not real tender except on the inside. But the outside is tough, and you will barely feel it.

FROM: jb

I inject into my stomach where the absorption is the fastest. Rotate the injection site or it will possibly start to form knots under the skin. My doctor checks my stomach at every visit to make sure that this is not happening.

Make sure the area you're going to use is clean. Your doctor may advise you to use alcohol to clean your skin. If you do, wait until the alcohol has evaporated before you inject or it will sting.

Your doctor or diabetes educator may tell you that you don't have to use alcohol and that soap-and-water cleaning is good enough. Some people inject through clothing, too. Discuss this option with your diabetes educator.

Be sure to inject at least two finger widths away from the last injection site, and don't inject yourself in the same place for at least a week. Don't inject near moles or scars.

Supplies

- A prepared and sterile syringe.

Instructions

1. Choose the location for the injection.
2. Push the needle straight into the skin. Don't move the syringe. Keep the needle straight.
3. Slowly (for a count of three to five) push the plunger in to inject the insulin.
4. Wait a few seconds for all of the insulin to go in. Remove the needle.
5. Cover the injection hole with your finger, dry cotton, or gauze and press down for five seconds. Don't rub.
6. Write down how much insulin you injected, the time and date, and the injection site.

SUBJECT: MY FIRST INJECTIONS

FROM: GH

Do I poke the entire needle into myself or just part of it? I've never done this before, so I have NO idea what I'm really doing here! I'm using the small needles. Mini-pen needles, I guess. They're the short ones.

FROM: im

I don't use a pen, I use syringe and vial, but with those you are supposed to insert the needle all the way in. I assume it's the same with the smaller pen needles. Good luck! It really doesn't feel like you think it's going to!

FROM: D3

Has the Dr given you any instruction? How to prep the site? Where to give it? The manufacturer of your pen(s) may have a website that includes a video demonstration of their use. When I had to take my first injection, it was with no instruction from my doc or anyone else, so I had to rely on the package insert from the box of syringes and what I could find online. Try doing a Google search under the name of whoever makes your pen. Again, good luck, and it's not as hard as it seems!

FROM: GH

Yeah, the nurse explained it, but I was sort of in "shock," so I didn't really catch it all.

FROM: hp1

Good luck. I think you'll be surprised at how little it hurts, but be ready for a big ol' adrenalin rush when you poke yourself for the first time! Once you do it a couple of times, it will become bbbooooorrring like the pills. Let us know how it goes.

FROM: GH

I did it. I gave myself my very first injection. I sat here, debating with myself for about five minutes, needle about half an inch away from my belly. And I sat there . . . sat there . . . sat there . . . and then,

I FINALLY poked that baby in there. All the way! I pressed the injection button, left it in for a slow count of five, and then took it out. Anyway, I'm gonna be an old hand at this before the day is done! Thanks for all your help, suggestions, and tips, everyone! It is greatly appreciated!

FROM: hp1
YAY! You did it! I so remember the sitting there with the needle poised and not being able to do it.

FROM: GH
I'm sure if someone was watching me, they'd have laughed their butt off! Talk about pathetic! But, it's not a problem at all! You have no idea how HAPPY that makes me!

SUBJECT: SHOOTING STYLES

FROM: lw11
When I first started, I would pinch the skin up and jab the needle in. Well try to jab it in . . . it would bounce off. Finally I realized that the simplest approach was: Pinch the skin just a little bit—not too tight or the needle will either bounce off or hurt a little bit. Place your finger on the plunger of the syringe and push the needle inward and the plunger downward once in the skin. It does not hurt and makes the nervousness go away after a few times doing it.

Reusing Syringes

Disposable syringes are designed for one use only, and manufacturers don't recommend reuse. Each time you use a needle, it gets duller and you'll feel it more. Still, many people do reuse syringes and have no problem.

However, if your skin isn't clean, you are ill, have open wounds on your hands, or have low resistance to infection, don't risk syringe reuse. If the needle touches anything other than clean skin, it's time to throw it away.

Instructions

1. Carefully recap the syringe.

2. Don't let the needle touch anything but clean skin and your insulin vial stopper. If it touches anything else, don't reuse it.
3. Store the used syringe at room temperature.
4. There will always be a tiny, even invisible, amount of insulin left in the syringe and needle. Use one syringe with just one type of insulin to avoiding mixing insulins.
5. Don't reuse a syringe in which you have mixed insulins. Some of the NPH might get into your rapid-acting insulin vial.
6. Don't reuse a needle that is bent or dull. But just because an injection is painful doesn't mean the needle is dull. You may have hit a nerve ending or have wet alcohol on your skin. Try a different spot. If it still hurts, use a new needle.
7. Don't wipe your needle with alcohol. This removes some of the coating that makes the needle go more smoothly into your skin.

SUBJECT: REUSE SYRINGES?

FROM: D

I used to use my syringes more than once, until I had to toss out over half a vial of insulin because it developed "floaties." I decided that buying a few extra syringes was worth a lot less than the hassle of getting another vial of insulin too early! I now believe in the "one time use" for syringes. I religiously use alcohol pads, too.

How to Dispose of Syringes and Pen Needles

Used syringes and needles are medical waste. Your town or county may have rules about throwing away needles and other medical waste such as lancets.

You can buy a device that clips and catches the syringe needle. Don't use scissors to clip off needle tips.

If you don't destroy the needles, recap them (if you can do it safely) and put them in a sharps container. You can buy these at your local pharmacy. Or use a non-see-through, heavy-duty plastic or metal container with a screw cap or tight lid. Label the container "MEDICAL WASTE—USED SHARPS." Don't use a container that will allow a needle to break through and possibly stick someone. Place the container in the trash, where it will not be confused with recycling.

SUBJECT: DISPOSAL

FROM: Mc

My doctor gave me a Humalog (lispro) pen this week. She advised me to change the needle every day. Can I just put the cap back on it and dispose of it as garbage or do I need to take special precautions with it?

FROM: gn

I place all my used needles, pens, and test strips in an old detergent bottle or juice bottle and screw the top on. Then I dispose of it (per my trash hauler's instructions). Or you can purchase a sharps container. My hauler lets me dispose of my needles and all in an old, sealed bottle.

FROM: cf
I use the pen as well and never reuse the needles. I do use a BD disposal thing. It is cheap, and it allows for easy disposal of the pen needles. I use this for my Byetta pen as well, and it uses the same needles.

OUT IN THE WORLD

You've done a trial injection in your diabetes educator's office. You've given yourself injections at home. Now, we hope, you're ready to get back to your life: shopping, eating out, and taking trips. Here's how others have incorporated insulin therapy into their daily lives.

SUBJECT: TESTING AND SYRINGING IN PUBLIC

FROM: lo18
How many people here test and syringe in public? Have you ever gotten told NOT to and/or kicked out or yelled at for doing so? I have both tested and injected in public, but I don't in front of children and parents, usually!

FROM: BA

In my personal and old-fashioned opinion, hygiene and medical procedures should not be performed in public if it is at all avoidable. They very especially should not be performed at a dining table. It is not that I'm squeamish. I just prefer a line preserved between public and private activity.

Having said that, I'll admit to testing in public once in a while. I've tried to make it as unobtrusive as possible, shielding what I was doing with a casually draped sweater. I never injected insulin in public in the several months I was on insulin. Perhaps if I was on it indefinitely I'd run into a situation where that was a necessity. We all do what we have to do and make the best of it. I vote for keeping testing and syringing out of public view.

FROM: Jm

I did my Lantus in Macy's once, and I had one lady look at me like I was crazy! I took my BS in a Longhorn steakhouse (in the bathroom, as I needed to wash hands), and the lady in there said it must be hard to test so much but that she was pre-diabetic after she had a stroke and did test at different times a day. Also met a nice older lady at Wendy's. She even said my number was great. I'm just waiting for someone to say something rude. I want to come back with a smartass comment like "I'm so glad your pancreas works!"

FROM: DL

I say you have to do what you have to do! If I am just testing to be testing, I usually wait until I am alone. Just a personal choice. But by all means, if I'm having a dizzy spell, out comes the meter and beep, pop, and I'm done. I just sit wherever I am a few minutes until I regain my composure and then I am fine.

FROM: D3

I will test in public if I feel like I am hypo. Otherwise, I will test in the car. I generally do not need to inject while in the open. That is one of the few advantages of using Reg insulin. It can take 30–45 minutes to start working and therefore allows me to take it in the car and not worry about how quickly the food will arrive.

FROM: d7

The polite thing to do is not test or "shoot up in public"—end of story. I don't want to risk upsetting or scaring a child. I take Byetta before a meal, and it's very easy to handle it in the car or in a restroom.

FROM: el0

I tested about a half hour [after lunch]. My BS was 331. Eeekkkk! So, we stopped on the side of the road to take my insulin, and a cop pulls up behind me just as I'm injecting! Holy crap, the cop was screaming, thought I was a druggy. I explained to him that I'm a diabetic injecting insulin. He didn't believe me, so he went through the whole ordeal of calling my doc's office and everything. It was crazy. I have a doc appt today, so I'm gonna pick up a paper explaining that I'm a diabetic to keep in my car.

FROM: Gnp
I test at the table and I take my insulin at the table. The meter is in my lap, so it's not obvious, and before I inject, I let everyone at the table know what I'm about to do. That way, they can look away. I always inject in a very private fashion—I'm using the sides of my tummy—and turn so that the rest of the world can't see me. That's standard procedure for me, though when we ate at Cracker Barrel and were right in the middle of the room and there wasn't any way to be subtle about it, I did wait until I was back in the car.

FROM: P2
I always test in the car before I go into a restaurant but that's a personal decision. I'm simply uncomfortable doing things like that in public. Maybe I'm a Puritan; who knows?

FROM: tia
I don't think we need to go off and hide to test or do shots. It's a part of our lives.

Index

Other Books from the American Diabetes Association

To order these and other great American Diabetes Association titles, call 1-800-232-6733 or visit *http://store.diabetes.org*. American Diabetes Association titles are also available in bookstores nationwide.

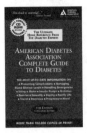

American Diabetes Association Complete Guide to Diabetes, 4th Edition
by American Diabetes Association
Have all the tips and information on diabetes that you need close at hand. The world's largest collection of diabetes self-care tips, techniques, and tricks for solving diabetes-related problems is bigger and better than ever before.
Order no. 4809-04; Price $29.95

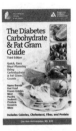

The Diabetes Carbohydrate & Fat Gram Guide, 3rd Edition
by Lea Ann Holzmeister, RD, CDE
Registered dietitian Lea Ann Holzmeister has put together complete nutritional information, including carbs, fat, calories, and more for nearly 7,000 listings. This new edition now features charts for fast foods and prepackaged meals.
Order no. 4708-03; Price $14.95

Diabetes Meal Planning Made Easy, 3rd Edition
by Hope S. Warshaw, MMSc, RD, CDE, BC-ADM
Let expert Hope Warshaw show you how to change unhealthy eating habits while continuing to enjoy the foods you love! Change your eating habits over time so that changes you make are the ones that last for life!
Order no. 4706-03; Price $14.95

Order online at *http://store.diabetes.org* or call toll-free at 1-800-232-6733.

About the American Diabetes Association

The American Diabetes Association is the nation's leading voluntary health organization supporting diabetes research, information, and advocacy. Its mission is to prevent and cure diabetes and to improve the lives of all people affected by diabetes. The American Diabetes Association is the leading publisher of comprehensive diabetes information. Its huge library of practical and authoritative books for people with diabetes covers every aspect of self-care—cooking and nutrition, fitness, weight control, medications, complications, emotional issues, and general self-care.

To order American Diabetes Association books: Call 1-800-232-6733 or log on to *http://store.diabetes.org*

To join the American Diabetes Association: Call 1-800-806-7801 or log on to *www.diabetes.org/membership*

For more information about diabetes or ADA programs and services: Call 1-800-342-2383. E-mail: AskADA@diabetes.org or log on to *www.diabetes.org*

To locate an ADA/NCQA Recognized Provider of quality diabetes care in your area: *www.ncqa.org/dprp*

To find an ADA Recognized Education Program in your area: Call 1-800-342-2383. *www.diabetes.org/for-health-professionals-and-scientists/recognition/edrecognition.jsp*

To join the fight to increase funding for diabetes research, end discrimination, and improve insurance coverage: Call 1-800-342-2383. *www.diabetes.org/advocacy-and-legalresources/advocacy.jsp*

To find out how you can get involved with the programs in your community: Call 1-800-342-2383. See below for program Web addresses.

American Diabetes Month: educational activities aimed at those diagnosed with diabetes—month of November. *www.diabetes.org/communityprograms-and-localevents/americandiabetesmonth.jsp*

American Diabetes Alert: annual public awareness campaign to find the undiagnosed—held the fourth Tuesday in March. *www.diabetes.org/communityprograms-and-localevents/americandiabetesalert.jsp*

American Diabetes Association Latino Initiative: diabetes awareness program targeted to the Latino community. *www.diabetes.org/communityprograms-and-localevents/latinos.jsp*

African American Program: diabetes awareness program targeted to the African American community. *www.diabetes.org/communityprograms-and-localevents/africanamericans.jsp*

Awakening the Spirit: Pathways to Diabetes Prevention & Control: diabetes awareness program targeted to the Native American community. *www.diabetes.org/communityprograms-and-localevents/nativeamericans.jsp*

To find out about an important research project regarding type 2 diabetes: *www.diabetes.org/diabetes-research/research-home.jsp*

To obtain information on making a planned gift or charitable bequest: Call 1-888-700-7029. *www.wpg.cc/stl/CDA/homepage/1,1006,509,00.html*

To make a donation or memorial contribution: Call 1-800-342-2383. *www.diabetes.org/support-the-cause/make-a-donation.jsp*

3 1143 00734 9732